FOR WARD BY KE

HORMONE Havoc

Dispelling the Myths & Misconceptions about Hormones in Women & Men

Terri DeNeui
DNP, APRN, ACNP-BC

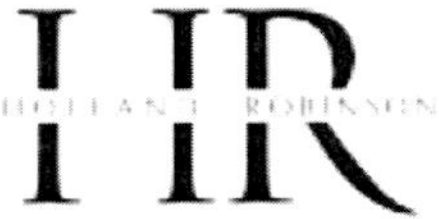

Holland Robinson Publishing

An imprint of Holland Robinson Publishing / Digging Up Dreams LLC

Fort Worth, Texas 76117

First Published in the United States of America by Holland Robinson Publishing 2023.

Book Design and Layout – Holland Robinson

Paperback ISBN: 978-1-961074-12-5

For more information, please visit

www.HollandRobinsonPublishing.com

or contact Info@HollandRobinsonPublishing.com.

PRAISE FOR HORMONE HAVOC!

I have had the pleasure to know Dr. Terri DeNeui since 2014, but it is only in the last 2-3 years that I have had the distinct privilege to teach and work alongside her on a regular basis.

Dr. DeNeui's knowledge about hormone therapy is unmatched, and her passion for the subject is obvious to anyone that has ever met her. Her approach to treating patients starts with listening, which is where all patient communication should start.

She has a commonsense approach that is backed by science and decades of experience. If every medical provider in the country would read this book and practice its teachings, the health and vitality of our country would change for the better.

In a nation where medicine is mired in sick care, disease management and polypharmacy, hormones are the foundation for well care, disease prevention and healthy aging.

Dr. DeNeui's dream is to make testosterone therapy standard of care for women. I share this goal. We are on a mission to change healthcare for the better, one patient at a time and one provider at a time.

This book is a gift to medical providers and to patients. Bravo Dr. DeNeui!

Johnny J Peet, M.D., FACOG

When I practiced and taught medicine, I concluded that medicine is an art informed by science. This book is a spectacular demonstration of that.

Dr. DeNeui's mastery of the art of treating the whole person enhanced by mastery of the science makes this book invaluable. Having been a hormone practitioner and patient, I found her book both informative and captivating. I couldn't put it down. I'm so glad this information is now available to people in such a coherent, readable format.

Peter P. Farmer, M.D.

Hormone Havoc is an eminently readable guide that aims to help us understand the crucial role of hormone optimization in supporting overall health and resilience. Through a compelling blend of scientific research, practical advice, and inspiring anecdotes, Terri DeNeui explains how harnessing the power of hormones elevates our well-being to new heights. Her passion for the subject shines through on every page. As she helps the reader navigate the intricate web of hormones, Terri DeNeui dispels decades-old myths while illuminating the profound influence of hormones on how we age. Hormone Havoc empowers individuals to take charge of their health journey by becoming their own hormone advocates, like the author herself.

The book catalyzes positive change, inspiring readers to make informed decisions and take proactive steps towards a life of vitality by saying "no" to a system that, through fear, misunderstanding, and misrepresentation, has led us down the road of low hormone complacency. As an outside-of-the-box neurologist who embraces brain health through hormone optimization, I will make this book essential reading for my patients whose greatest desire is to restore the health in healthcare.

Kenneth S. Sharlin, M.D., M.P.H., IFMCP
Founder, The Brain Tune Up! Program
Sharlin Health and Neurology, LLC

Hormone Havoc is the kind of book more doctors need to write! Three things are immediately evident as you engage this important work.

First, it is clear that Dr. DeNeui thinks differently about the human body. Rather than throw drugs at a diagnosis, she seems to see the body as capable of its own well-being when given the keys to function as it is designed. Second, she has made it easy for me, a non-medical professional to understand my own body. Third and perhaps most important, she cares.

It is clear that she cares that you and I feel better and that we regain the fullness of life for which we were designed. This book will help you and the truth in this book will help you even more!

Bob Hamp LMFT
Therapist, Author, Speaker, Co-Founder of Think Differently Academy

Dr. Terri DeNeui, a trusted friend and accomplished practitioner, expertly intertwines scientific depth with reader-friendly accessibility in her groundbreaking exploration of hormone therapy. With a deep understanding of the subject matter, she effortlessly distills complex concepts into easily comprehensible insights.

By addressing true deficiencies within the body, Dr. DeNeui empowers individuals from all walks of life to embark on a transformative journey towards a more vibrant and fulfilling existence. With her invaluable guidance, you can unlock the secrets to optimal hormone health and embrace a life of vitality.

Dr. Jon Chasteen,

Author and Pastor, Victory Church OKC & Grapevine Texas

Terri DeNeui is a practitioner that is on a never-ending quest to provide the best possible care for her patients and is committed to searching for solutions that make it happen. This book is a clear example of the commitment to excellence and passion for sharing her knowledge to help people with their journey back to health.

Jim LaValle,

Clinical Pharmacist, CCN, MT, DHM, DHPh
Author & Founder of The Metabolic Code

DEDICATION

For everyone who has been plagued with a health issue, sought answers in many places and from many people, only to think you must be crazy because all you've been told is "you are normal, nothing is wrong", this book is for you.

ACKNOWLEDGEMENTS

This book has been a journey 15 years in the making, a labor of love….and fear, and laughter, and confusion, and hope - I guess I just described life!

My highest praises and gratitude are to God for gifting me with the "need to know", the ability to teach what I know effectively, and for protecting me along the way.

The thousands of patients who have taught me so much, simply because they trusted me enough to ask questions to which I had to find answers.

The incredible staff and leadership at EVEXIAS Medical Centers. I could not have gotten this done without such an amazing team keeping the ship thriving in my absence, each one of you is an integral part of what this book is about.

The amazing corporate staff, practitioners, and teaching faculty of EVEXIAS Health Solutions. What you do every day is exceptional and important! On days it feels overwhelming, don't forget the impact you have on the lives you are positively changing.

Dr. Johnny Peet, chairman of EVEXIAS Health Solutions Medical Board, exceptional co-leader, and educator of our clinical trainings. Your commitment to the endeavor of changing healthcare is appreciated beyond words. Your passion for teaching is palpable and infectious. I am honored to work alongside you!

A few key mentors whom I have learned a great deal over the years that caused me to see the beautiful systems of the human body in new and different ways:

Dr. Neal Rouzier, you are a pioneer in the hormone space. Working with you over the past decade changed my clinical practice because of your passion in challenging the status quo that is Western medicine - "association doesn't prove causation".

Dr. Jim LaValle, when I listened to you speak for the first time seven years ago about the gut, nutrition, and peptides, I remember wishing I could live in your brain for a week! I would have never dreamed I would have the privilege to work alongside you changing the paradigm of healthcare. Understanding the body as a "system of systems" is a key concept I have never forgotten and has radically changed the way I approach health concerns with my patients.

Bob Hamp, I am eternally grateful for the ways you have challenged me to Think Differently (not different!). Your nonjudgmental listening and ways you have taught me to approach the world around me have been invaluable.

The ripple effect of your gifts on my life- my marriage, my family, my profession, our companies, and staff - will last for generations to come.

Last, but never least, Captain Crash- what a ride this has been! You inspire me in many ways, but the most important is to always ask myself how I can be better. None of it would have been possible, or as much fun, without you, DDD! I am so grateful for that serendipitous plane ride on August 14, 2009. All my love, Your Beauty Queen.

FOREWORD

In this compelling and enlightening book, Dr. Terri DeNeui invites us to embark on a transformative journey — one that is guided by her remarkable tenderness, profound knowledge, and unwavering courage. Terri's path has been one less traveled, venturing into realms where others have often feared to go. Through her experiences, she has emerged as a beacon of understanding and a source of profound insight into a subject that is both complicated and complex.

Terri's dedication to the full integration of body, mind, and spirit is unparalleled. As a renowned practitioner and visionary, she has cultivated a deep understanding of the intricate connections within the human experience. In her pursuit of knowledge, she has fearlessly explored the uncharted territories of holistic healthcare, drawing upon the wisdom of both ancient traditions and cutting-edge research. The result is a wealth of information that she shares with us in these pages — a treasure trove of wisdom that will illuminate our path and empower us to reclaim our well-being.

In the course of my own journey, I have worked with various practitioners, each contributing their unique expertise. However, it is Terri DeNeui who has left an indelible mark on my life. Through her EVEXIAS clinics and the EVEXIAS healthcare providers she has trained, she has fostered places where individuals can find solace and healing, allowing them to transcend the chaos of "hormone havoc" and discover what I call *"hormone harmony"*.

Kelly Le Brock

Actor, Philanthropist, Women's Health Advocate

PREFACE

"The greatest medicine of all is teaching people how not to need it."
Hippocratées

This is one of my favorite quotes from Hippocrates. It is foundational to how I approach patient care and what I teach the practitioners who come to the training company I lead, hoping to do more for their patients and rediscover their passion for healing. Healthcare providers have been trained to prescribe medications that primarily only treat the symptoms. When educating healthcare providers on how to change their mindset and create a paradigm shift from a "symptom-based treatment model" to a "root cause discovery model," this quote from Hippocrates is where I begin.

Have you ever found yourself tired all the time, sad or moody, not being able to think or focus well, not sleeping through the night, having random aches and pains or joint pain when you wake up, or being challenged with maintaining a healthy weight? Have you ever gone to your healthcare provider with some (or all) of these complaints, only to be given a prescription for an antidepressant, an anxiety medication, a sleeping pill, or be told you just need to eat less and exercise more? Have you ever filled those prescription medications and found that your symptoms didn't improve much, or you had side effects like more weight gain or not feeling like yourself? Or have you had some of these issues and sought medical help, only to be told you're "normal" or "your labs are normal," and "you are just under too much stress"? (That actually translates as, "I don't know what is wrong with you, but here is a prescription that may help your symptoms.")

Well, I understand completely! Not only have I experienced many of these symptoms myself, but thousands of patients have come to me—or one of the many healthcare providers I have trained—with these exact complaints. The good news is, there is usually a root cause that is quite easy to treat.

I am a clinically trained and certified, doctoral-prepared adult acute care nurse practitioner with a passion for understanding the "why" behind many questions related to the human body, health, and disease. I always wanted to be a medical doctor, but as a young single mother at the age of 19, working as a cake decorator and assistant manager of a local grocery store, making $5.25 an hour, the registered nurse (RN) track was a quicker way to develop a career and start making enough money to support my small family.

The desire to understand "why" every time a doctor at the hospital would write an order or prescribe a medication often got me in trouble — those doctors did not like being questioned. I felt it was my duty to understand what I was doing and why so that I could rest assured I was indeed doing what was best for the patient. As the years have passed, relationships between doctors and nurses have changed, and most physicians appreciate and respect the nurses who ask why, especially when it is done from a space of curiosity and not superiority.

My thirst for knowledge fuels my ongoing quest to learn more and fueled my desire to expand my education. From a registered nurse (RN) to a nurse practitioner working in a hospital setting to opening my own clinic and ultimately obtaining my clinical doctorate degree, this drive pushes me to continuously seek the latest clinical studies for my patients and colleagues. It inspires me to never stop asking questions—sometimes the same question repeatedly because with new and emerging research, the next answer could change a patient's life!

The doctoral pursuit gave me the tools and insights into the research process, allowing me to research, write and publish papers of my own, as well as create evidence-based lectures to share with other healthcare providers, so they might offer their own patients a path to an improved, healthier life as free from disease as possible.

The term disease can be understood simply by examining the root of the word dis-ease. We have come to think of disease as tangible illness like heart disease, cancer, and the like. However, when you take step back and examine a person as a whole being, dis-ease manifests from and/or in three primary forms: *the mind, the body, and the spirit (or soul).* Although this book is primarily focused on the physical aspects of disease and prevention thereof, simultaneously nurturing the mind and spirit cannot be ignored when trying to achieve optimal health and wellness.

My journey from cake decorator to nurse to doctoral prepared nurse practitioner to clinic practice owner, researcher, lecturer, and author was not easy, but it has never really felt like work. You know what they say, when you love what you do and are operating in your gifts, it doesn't feel like work. Humans are unique beings. Each of us are born with distinctive gifts and a calling on our lives, and whole-body wellness is fundamental to ensuring a lifetime of sharing those gifts with others in our sphere of influence.

"Humans are unique beings. Each of us are born with distinctive gifts and a calling on our lives, and whole-body wellness is fundamental to ensuring a lifetime of sharing those gifts with others in our sphere of influence."

My passion is teaching people the importance of and how to optimize health in every area- mind, body, and spirit - so the calling on their lives may be shared with the world for a lifetime.

How did I make the paradigm shift from my training as a prescription writer for symptoms to root cause analyzer of disease?

It was my third night shift in a row at a busy emergency room of a large Metroplex hospital in the Dallas-Fort Worth area. Patient after patient presenting to the emergency room during those 36 hours had consequences of some chronic disease process. A 57-year-old male with a heart attack secondary to coronary artery disease, a 53-year-old male with complications of uncontrolled type 2 diabetes, a 70-year-old female who suffered a fracture from a fall secondary to osteoporosis, a 65-year-old female with new onset of stroke symptoms, a postpartum female on suicide watch for severe postpartum depression, a 55-year-old female with severe anxiety and a panic attack that she thought was a heart attack, a 61-year-old female with complications of a radiation treatment for breast cancer, and a 72-year-old female with early onset Alzheimer's dementia.

I remember thinking to myself, "The vast majority of the patients I've seen the past three days all have preventable chronic diseases that are causing their admission to the hospital. Why aren't we doing more for prevention?" As an emergency room nurse, and subsequently an acute care nurse practitioner, I was attracted to the adrenaline rush of working in a busy emergency department. "Saving lives is where it's at!" I remember when I embarked on my journey to higher education, I thought, "I never want to work in a primary care office, how boring!" At 2 a.m. on that last stretch of a 36-hour run, I had an epiphany: there has to be a better way to prevent emergency issues rooted in chronic disease and allow patients and their families to live healthy, exuberant lives!

"There has to be a better way to prevent emergency issues rooted in chronic disease and allow patients and their families to live healthy, exuberant lives!"

And so, my journey began. I had no idea where it would lead me. I had to uncover other ways to approach treating disease processes because the current standard of care—then and now—does nothing to prevent chronic diseases. I started a small clinic in a 10 x 10 suite while I continued to work weekends at the hospital. I partnered with another practitioner who was starting a weight loss clinic, and when a local pharmacist invited me to a conference—all expenses paid—to learn more about hormones and their impact on health, I was intrigued.

Now, if I'm being totally honest, I was more excited about an all-expenses-paid first-class trip to Las Vegas than I was about a hormone conference. I never had any interest in hormones. In fact, at the time, I thought I was much too young to be worrying about hormones and "the change" discussed in hushed tones among women over 50. I had no idea that the stigma of menopause and andropause, a.k.a. midlife crisis in men, was no laughing matter but a key insight into the role hormones play in chronic disease prevention. During that conference, while sitting in a lecture listening to a doctor describe the life change in her patients on hormone therapy, I had a moment of clarity, really a Divine whisper, telling me this is what I am supposed to do.

CONTENTS

CHAPTER 1

INTRODUCTION

"Hormones get no respect. We think of them as the elusive chemicals that make us a bit moody, but these magical little molecules do so much more."
Susannah Cahalan

In 2008, when I began the journey of opening my own clinic, I never imagined that my pursuits would elevate me to my position today. I am honored to be a key thought leader in the field of hormone optimization and preventive medicine and an educator that supports practitioners in discovering a whole new way to practice medicine and truly transform the lives of their patients.

I could not have imagined patient after patient walking into my office that were like 65-year-old Bobbie. She arrived in my office when her 78-year-old husband, a retired gynecologist, came to me desperately seeking help for her.

You see, his daughter was my patient as well. Six months prior, when she arrived in my office, her marriage was on the rocks, but her treatment plan completely changed her life. She came to realize that all the years of discord and malcontent in her marriage were primarily from her own misery rooted in hormone decline. The prescriptions she was on didn't help; in fact, they made some things worse. The antidepressant that was prescribed caused her to gain weight, her libido was non-existent, and although she wasn't necessarily "moody and depressed," she was emotionally apathetic. Her children and husband felt these medications made her worse, not better. When I got her off those medications and optimized her hormones, the root cause of her low libido, weight gain, and emotional apathy was addressed. The clarity that came with her treatment plan allowed her to recognize the same misery in her own mother, whom she prodded to come see me. *She finally did.*

I have to say, I was somewhat intimidated. I knew I was going to get quite a few questions from this gynecologist husband regarding what I did, considering gynecologists are assumed to be the key providers and thought leaders of hormone care. He was at a loss, however. A decade prior, he had put his wife on the usual synthetic hormone combination of an estrogen and progestin, but after the release of the Women's Health Initiative (WHI) trial results, he, like tens of thousands of other doctors and patients across the country, stopped his wife's hormones and stopped prescribing hormones to his patients. There was an unfounded fear that hormone therapy in women would cause strokes, Alzheimer's disease, osteoporosis, heart attacks and breast cancer.

Armed with a great deal of knowledge and a plethora of medical studies, I was ready to answer all his questions and challenges. But that never came to pass. Once I assessed her, reviewed her bloodwork, and developed a treatment plan to optimize her hormones, they were all in. *He was desperately seeking answers.*

Four weeks later, Bobbie was back in my office getting her aftercare lab work. I walked up to say hello and ask how she was doing. She immediately started crying, and I thought, "Uh-oh, I must have gotten this one wrong!" Once she regained her composure, she said, "I have not liked my husband for 25 years! …. And now I realize it was me and not him." She went on to share how sad she was at the loss of time, and she felt like she did not have much time left with him to enjoy her newfound vitality, joy, zeal for life, and, of course, sex drive!

Two weeks later, I walked in to see my next patient, and lo and behold, it was the good doctor, husband of Bobbie! When I sat down, he said, "Before you get started, I want to thank you for giving me my wife back." He choked up a bit and went on to say, "Had I known about this therapy when I was a practicing gynecologist, based on the changes I've seen in my wife and daughter, I would've put every single female on it. Now," he continued with a sly smile, "I am here to get your therapy for myself so I can keep up with her!" You see, he also was lamenting the loss of time — time wasted not knowing how to care for his hormonally depleted wife and patients when he was in clinical practice.

Hormone optimization is not just for women! I have thousands of stories of male patients complaining of a decreased zest for life, including the inability to focus and concentrate at work, joint pain, irritability, food cravings, weight gain, or lack of desire to engage in things they love, like hunting, fishing, or golfing. With treatment—at my clinic or at the clinic of one of the now thousands of providers I, and other amazing teachers, have trained nationwide—these men rediscover life when their hormones are optimized. And not to mention, many of the women who experience hormone optimization are quickly followed by their husbands because without hormone balance, he can no longer keep up with her zest, energy, and sex drive!

In particular, one male patient, a well-known speaker, author, and thought leader in his field was referred to me by another patient. I remember when he sat down in my office the first thing he said to me was, "I'm ready to retire. I just don't have it in me to keep doing what I'm doing. So, no pressure," he said, "but this better work!" I reviewed his extensive lab tests, as well as a detailed medical history, and discovered not only was his testosterone low, but his thyroid was very low, and he had gut issues that were causing a great deal of inflammation and likely contributing to his depression. More on the gut-brain connection later.

His treatment plan included all hormone optimization-testosterone, thyroid, DHEA and melatonin - and key dietary changes. When I saw him four weeks later to review his follow-up lab tests and discuss how he was feeling, he couldn't believe how much energy he had and his exuberance for life had returned. He exclaimed his gratitude and said "I was almost ready to throw in the towel, but this therapy gave me back my passion and drive. I still have so much more to give and share with the world!"

I can tell you story after story of people whose lives were changed when they experienced hormone optimization: couples who were on the brink of divorce ripping up divorce papers or women who struggled with depression for over a decade after the birth of their last child—all suddenly resolved without anti-anxiety medications, antidepressants, or sleeping pills. Or the type 2 diabetics who no longer require daily medication because after hormone optimization, they have increased energy and stamina, as well as decreased cholesterol and cortisol, and subsequently, insulin resistance. Or the chronic menstrual migraine patient who had been to multiple doctors, including neurologist, and on multiple medications to no avail, who, within four weeks of her first testosterone treatment noted her migraines had stopped completely!

I can tell you stories of breast cancer survivors who were told they could never have hormones again, leaving them feeling hopeless and subjected to a life of misery. However, after working with me, or one of the practitioners in our nationwide network, are now living a full life because of testosterone therapy. Our providers understand that testosterone is a vital female hormone, shown in clinical studies to be breast protective and may even prevent breast cancer!

"Our providers understand that testosterone is a vital female hormone, shown in clinical studies to be breast protective and may even prevent breast cancer!"

I can share stories of couples who had not been intimate for decades because after the wife transitioned through menopause, it hurt too much to have intercourse, not to mention the lack of desire.

I can share story after story of chronic pain sufferers whose diminished quality of life was only further exacerbated by hormonal decline, secondary to their pain and medication regimen. Some of these same patients were unable to walk upstairs without agonizing pain, but after just two weeks on the right form and doses hormone therapy, these patients reported that their joint pain was completely gone.

"The U.S. performs poorly on most measures of health compared to other high-income countries."

According to the American Public Health Association (APHA), the U.S. performs poorly on most measures of health compared to other high-income countries. Study after study shows the U.S. spends more on health care but has worse health outcomes across age, gender, and income groups than comparable countries around the world. Why is that, and what can be done about it? It is my fervent hope that by the end of this book, you can start making some inferences for yourself about what to do about it.

First and foremost: Ask why! Why am I being given this prescription for a medication, a lab or diagnostic test, or advice on how to treat a problem? Is the root cause of my depression a selective serotonin reuptake inhibitor (SSRI), medication like Prozac, deficiency? Is the root cause of my sleepless nights an Ambien deficiency? Is the root cause of my anxiety a Xanax deficiency? Is the root cause of my inability to focus, or "adult ADD" a deficiency of a central nervous system stimulant like Concerta or Aderall? I could give dozens of examples like this, but you get my point. Don't get me wrong; many of these medications have been life savers for many people during times of crisis, but that is exactly what most medications are intended for: a temporary solution to the symptoms of *a problem while the root cause is being addressed. Many medications were not intended for lifelong use to Band-aid a symptom.* Unfortunately, that is where many of us find ourselves - perpetually on medications that are not fixing the problem, and what's worse, many of them cause other problems you may need another prescription for!

"Medications are intended for a temporary solution to the symptoms of a problem while the root cause is being addressed."

This book will take you on a journey that provides key information dispelling myths about sex hormone therapy for men and women, but also an exploration of additional key hormones and nutrients that play a role in whole body wellness.

CHAPTER 2

THE HORMONES

The word hormone (hormon root) in Greek means "that which sets in motion" or "to impel, urge on." This definition of the root of the word makes perfect sense when you understand the symptoms of inadequate hormone(s) in your body. The feeling is the exact opposite of "set in motion" or "impel." You experience sluggishness, fatigue, depressed mood, depressed affect, lack of joy, lack of vitality for life, lack of optimal cellular function, which can lead to inflammation, which leads to many chronic diseases and pain.

Hormone receptors are present on literally every single cell in the human body from head to toe! They are chemical messengers that travel from one part of the body to other parts of the body and help control how certain cells and organs do their work, "setting in motion" the intended function of that cellular system. When there are no chemical messengers available to "impel" the actions of those cells, degeneration, decline, and disease begins.

"But wait," you may ask, "I thought hormones were just for hot flashes in women and erectile function in men? What is all this talk of young women, testosterone and depression, young men with symptoms of testosterone deficiency?" Indeed, symptoms of hormone imbalance may start younger than you think.

Most women start feeling the decline in their testosterone levels after their second child. Young women on birth control pills also feel testosterone decline because of the increase in sex hormone-binding globulin, a protein that binds up free testosterone, leading to low levels of free testosterone and the appearance of symptoms.

More and more young men are presenting with testosterone deficiency. Why is such extreme hormonal decline in young men being seen? The primary cause is thought to be endocrine disruption due to chemicals and hormone - like substances in our environment, including our food supply, the air, chemicals in clothing, bedding and furniture, and a myriad of other "assaults" to our bodies.

The point of all this is that hormone decline deserves attention well before the fifth decade of life for both men and women. There are a variety of reasons that hormone insufficiency occurs at much younger ages and stages of life. It is pertinent the general population and healthcare providers understand that feeling depressed, anxious, irritable, sleepless nights, lack of focus, chronic pain, and sexual dysfunction are

"Feeling depressed, anxious, irritable, sleepless nights, lack of focus, chronic pain, and sexual dysfunction are not normal, and there is a root cause."

not normal, and there is a root cause. The root cause certainly isn't a deficiency of an antidepressant, sleeping pill, anxiety pill, or attention deficit disorder (ADD) medication! The root cause is often hormonal decline and/or deficiency of key nutrients involved in hormone production, hormone receptor activity, and hormone metabolism

For the sake of discussion, the sex hormones referred to are testosterone, estrogen, and progesterone. Other very important hormones for overall body functioning and chronic disease prevention are DHEA, melatonin, and the thyroid hormones. Key aspects of hormone function, metabolism, and receptor site activity such as gut health and certain nutrients will also be explained. At the end of this book, references related to each topic discuss will be provided.

Before I get into a discussion about each hormone, where they come from, and the importance of each in the different body systems, it's vital to understand where the fear of sex hormones and sex hormone therapy originated—most notably the unfounded fear that hormones will cause breast cancer, strokes, heart attacks, and/or dementia in women.

"The WHI for hormone replacement therapy (HRT) standards is a dead and irrelevant paradigm to modern HRT that needs to be buried."
Marie Hoäg, MBA

HOW DID THIS HAPPEN?

Tens of thousands of men and women suffering from suboptimal hormones are left untreated. Why is that? Why do healthcare providers reach for the prescription pad and write out prescriptions for antidepressants, sleeping pills, or anxiety pills as a first line of defense? Or to be more natural in their approach, why do practitioners advise their patients to eat less and exercise more? Although that is an excellent recommendation, when people are suffering from extreme fatigue, depression, mood swings, irritability, inability to focus, and sleeplessness the last thing on their mind is altering dietary habits or getting to the gym to work out!

Why is no one looking at hormone insufficiency or deficiency as a root cause of common complaints and ailments? Men and women both suffer from these symptoms, as well as decreased vitality, loss of muscle mass, increased belly fat, and chronic pain, to name a few. Notice I didn't mention low sex drive, erectile dysfunction, or hot flashes? Those are a given; most people understand those issues are usually hormone related, but the other common complaints—more often than not—go largely ignored. My opinion, from training thousands of healthcare providers over the past 12 years, is because practitioners are simply not taught these concepts in medical training or advanced practice programs. Further, because these things are not taught, the alternative is biased education from drug companies and / or clinical practice guidelines that are often based on "expert opinion" and misinterpreted medical studies.

The WHI

Time Magazine, July 22, 2002, front cover: <u>The Truth About Hormones: Hormone replacement therapy is riskier than advertised. What's a woman to do?</u>

The above headline showcases the line in the sand: the point in time when hormones became this big scary thing for millions of women and their practitioners. The media loves to put a negative spin on things, doesn't it? *Scary headlines sell!*

And when the headlines are wide and far-reaching people take action—sometimes, perhaps often, without merit. In this case, women tossed their hormone therapy, and healthcare providers quit prescribing the therapy all together. At this point in time, no one investigated the truth. Everyone, it seemed, just reacted to the news. *Sound familiar?*

Unfortunately, tens of thousands of women died needlessly as a direct result of stopping their hormones, or never starting them at all. This unfounded fear was induced by media hype, like the aforementioned Time Magazine article, and misinformation around the Women's Health Initiative trial.

The Women's Health Initiative trial, also known as the WHI, was largest research trial to date on women and hormone therapies. Much has been gleaned from the subsequent data of the WHI over the last two decades, but the initial research results that were reported had devastating consequences. The trial was divided between two groups: women who had had hysterectomies (uterus removed) and women who had not. Hysterectomized women were placed on an equine (horse) estrogen product called Premarin. Women who had no hysterectomy, were placed on a Premarin and progestin combination called PremPro. The progestin, often erroneously referred to as progesterone, in the PremPro combination medication must not be confused with natural progesterone. More on this later in the chapter about progesterone.

The trial began in 1991 and was to end in 2005. The primary intention of the trial was to prove that estrogen hormone replacement therapy was preventive for heart attacks and death. Clinicians across the country had seen benefit in their female patients regarding the prevention of cardiovascular disease when they were on Premarin. The secondary intention of the trial was to examine the safety of the therapy as it pertained to invasive breast cancer risk and determine the impact of hormone therapy on osteoporosis. The trial came to an abrupt halt in 2002 because the invasive breast cancer risk in the PremPro group exceeded the boundaries for safety.

The PremPro, or estrogen and progestin combination, arm of the trial showed a significant increased risk of breast cancer, heart disease, Alzheimer's disease, and strokes. The Premarin only, or estrogen only, arm of the trial showed *protection* against breast cancer, Alzheimer's disease, cardiovascular disease, osteoporosis, and colorectal cancer. Unfortunately for an innumerable number of women across the country, the results were reported in such a way that bundled all hormone therapies under one umbrella. Rather than reporting the two separate arms of the trial, the media promoted all hormones as dangerous medications that caused heart attack and breast cancer and advised women to flush their hormones down the toilet immediately! At the same time, prescribers were advised to stop prescribing at once!

And that is exactly what happened .

Clinical practice guidelines, documents that most clinicians follow regarding treatment of a certain problems, changed drastically based on the initial results of the WHI. Health policy decisions were also affected by the confusion around the reported results of the trial. Before the WHI, it was standard belief that estrogen hormone therapy was heart and bone protective. After the trial, however, guidelines and public policy changed. Rather than taking a closer look at the design of the study, including the selected drugs, trial subjects, and data, a collective, knee-jerk conclusion was made: hormones are bad, and no one should take them, but if you do, you absolutely must stop by age 60.

Other guidelines stated that women should only take the lowest possible dose for the shortest amount of time and no more than five years. An important thing to understand about the study's flawed design is that a significant portion of the women in the trial were of advanced age, over 70, and had never been on hormones; many had pre-existing chronic diseases like hypertension and cardiovascular disease, and over 30 percent of the patients were considered clinically obese. Mind you, this does not represent the average woman presenting for menopausal hormone therapy.

The biggest failure of the WHI reports was the classification of all hormone therapies and medications as the same, with the same clinical outcomes. Today, researchers, scientists, and

"The biggest failure of the WHI reports was the classification of all hormone therapies and medications as the same, with the same clinical outcomes."

practitioners continue to unravel this web of misinformation. Sadly, as one major study reported, the number of excess deaths in women ages 50-59 who had a hysterectomy and avoided hormones exceeded 91,000 over a 10-year period. That was just women ages 50-59 who had a hysterectomy, not to mention post-menopausal women with a uterus or older post-menopausal women who avoided hormones out of fear from misinterpreted information! Then, in 2020, a key article in the Journal of American Medical Association (JAMA) touted estrogen not only to be protective against breast cancer, but also protect from death because of breast cancer (breast cancer mortality). More on this later when I talk about estrogen and breast cancer. So why isn't TIME Magazine creating a new headline showing the positive benefits of estrogen for women and reversing the misinformation about breast cancer and estrogen? Why aren't they recanting the old headline that started all the nonsense in the first place? Unfortunately, positive news doesn't sell. It's almost criminal in my opinion.

The impact of misinterpreted research affects men too. The primary method in which practitioners prescribe testosterone to males is based on a guideline established by the Endocrine Society. This guideline is quite cumbersome in that it requires a healthcare provider to test a male's testosterone level at 8 a.m. on two separate occasions. If the total testosterone level comes back as less than 300, that clinician is advised—not required—to follow an algorithm that takes the patient and clinician down an unnecessary path to first exclude reversible illnesses or nutritional deficiencies and then repeat the lab. If the testosterone is still less than 300, look at other possible issues and labs for other pituitary hormones and possibly an

MRI and maybe add a test for a rare genetic defect called Klinefelter syndrome.

Nowhere in the clinical practice guidelines does it recommend that the prescriber treat the patient's symptoms of low testosterone and ascertain if his clinical complaints resolve. The other unnecessary lab and diagnostic tests are possibly beneficial in a very young male, teens to 20s, who you would not expect to have a testosterone of less than 300, but certainly not in the average male who presents to a clinician's office with these symptoms.

It has been well documented in the clinical literature that male testosterone levels fall by up to 10 percent per year starting at age 35, and that percentage of decrease accelerates after age 40 and even more after age 50. The other aspect not being considered in this guideline is the availability of the patient's *free* testosterone.

Free testosterone is the most important number to look at in both males and females. Many people can have a total testosterone in the "normal range" and have several variables that prevent conversion to free testosterone, as well as receptor site resistance, which is not measurable on any laboratory marker. Don't get me wrong. I believe modern medicine and the diagnostic tools available are very beneficial, and looking for a root cause of a health complaint is imperative in most cases, but often, when it comes to hormone therapies, practitioners should stop looking for "zebras on Greene Street," meaning stop looking for an exotic diagnosis when something more obvious is evident and can be effectively treated.

WHAT ARE "NORMAL" HORMONE LEVELS?

I get this question as a clinician and as an educator regularly. Diagnostic tools, while highly valuable, tend to operate on averages and cookie-cutter scenarios, leading to treatment plans that are not tailored to the unique needs of each individual. Each human is an individual with many different variables that can influence not only hormone production but also hormone receptor activity, hormone metabolism, and excretion of those metabolites.

"Each human is an individual with many different variables that can influence not only hormone production but also hormone receptor activity, hormone metabolism, and excretion of those metabolites."

It's what I call the "art of medicine." Healthcare providers should be examining each patient as a total individual and not just a piece of paper with a snapshot of whatever is floating around their blood at that moment in time, and certainly not comparing that individual's blood test to society as a whole, which is where most clinical reference ranges originate.

Often, patients will bring me their lab test from another provider with the comment, "I was told my labs are normal," yet they haven't been given answers to why they feel so terrible. My answer to that statement is simple: *"Normal is not always optimal."*

When you look at lab reference ranges, especially as it relates to the different hormones the human body produces, that reference range is based on the average of a relatively unhealthy population; further, it's a bell-curve average. I share with my patients, "Wouldn't you always want to be on the right side of the bell curve?", meaning above average. If you were in school and studying for a test, are you shooting for the lowest score or the left side of the bell curve average? Usually not. It shouldn't be that way with our health either! The right side of the bell curve, or the upper end of a reference range on a lab value, is what I consider "optimal." The "right side" of the lab reference range is also what has correlated with my patients and patients of practitioners in our nationwide network feeling the best. We develop a treatment plan designed to move patients from the left side of the bell curve where they are in the "normal reference range" but experiencing every symptom of hormone insufficiency (including thyroid) all the way to the right side of the bell curve, the optimal side, where the patient's symptoms "magically" resolve.

For those who are data junkies like me, there is an abundance of clinical studies that speak to the lack of evidence that absolute blood hormone levels correlate with symptom presentation. If there is one clear message I hope you get from reading this book, it is that hormone therapy, in the correct forms and doses is safe and effective and, like thousands of my patients would attest, could very well change your life for the better!

CHAPTER 3

ESTROGEN

"I've seen estrogen make princesses out of witches."
Marie Hoäg, MBA

"The goal is to get your estrogen where it should be, so you don't have to hang out in social support groups that do nothing but chew the cud on how miserable they are without estrogen."
Marie Hoäg, MBA

Poor estrogen, it always gets a bad rap! Estrogen was the golden child of hormones in the middle part of the twentieth century, when clinicians were prescribing the "miracle drug" Premarin I spoke of earlier, and seeing women literally come back to life. They also observed this magical hormone restored vitality and moods and had a profoundly positive impact on the prevention of cardiovascular disease. Unfortunately, since the early 2000s, after the misconstrued results of the WHI were released to the public, estrogen has been blamed for everything, from cancer to heart attacks to strokes and everything in between!

A physician colleague of mine, Dr. Johnny Peet, often leads his lectures asking, "What if the WHI used natural estrogen (estradiol) and natural progesterone instead of synthetic Premarin and synthetic progestin (PremPro)?" This is an excellent question.

I believe that if doctors, scientists, and researchers of that study had used natural (bio-identical)—or as close to natural to human hormones as you can get—the study would have produced vastly different results. Imagine the diseases that could have been prevented, like osteoporosis, cardiovascular disease, and yes, even breast cancer! Imagine the deaths that could have been prevented from falls secondary to osteoporosis, cardiovascular disease, and Alzheimer's disease. Imagine the relationships that could have been salvaged as a woman transitioned through menopause feeling truly crazy, sometimes sadly suicidal and/or homicidal! The peri-menopausal woman often expresses outwardly these confused emotions towards those she loves most: her spouse, her family, and often her friends and coworkers. Not to mention all of the women who have suffered over the past two decades after being refused this vital hormone! All these things might have been prevented for tens of thousands of women, simply by using the right medication in one of the largest studies on women's health to date.

However, let's take it one step further: what if the study continued, and researchers also looked at the impact of testosterone on women's health? This is yet another incredibly powerful hormone the female ovaries make that plays a vital role in depression and mood, libido and overall sense of well-being. Testosterone was studied in the mid-1940s in women who had had their ovaries removed, and the results were astounding when they combined it with estrogen. Everything was better when testosterone was added to the hormone therapy regime! Why isn't testosterone in women studied more? The answer is simple. There is no pharmaceutical drug, or synthetic testosterone being marketed for women. At one time a synthetic drug called methyl testosterone was utilized in postmenopausal women, but it showed an increased risk of breast and uterine cancer rates due to the conversion to an estrogen hormone metabolite that is more carcinogenic (cancer causing). It has since been taken off the market in the states, and no other testosterone drugs for women have been researched or developed by the pharmaceutical industry. More on testosterone in women later.

WHO NEEDS ESTROGEN?

"Everyone needs estrogen! Estrogen is not just about hot flashes; it plays a vital role in all major organ systems in women and men!"

Well, everyone needs estrogen! Estrogen is not just about hot flashes; it plays a vital role in all major organ systems in women and men! Yes, that's right, men too! Just like women need testosterone, at lower levels of course, men make and need estrogen for sexual health, libido, prevention of metabolic syndrome (type 2 diabetes, obesity, and high blood pressure) and heart health.

Estrogen prevents coronary artery disease and has also been shown in studies to prevent strokes as well as protecting the area of injury after a stroke or heart attack, mitigating damage because it is a powerful anti-inflammatory molecule. The body converts massive amounts of estrogen via an enzyme called aromatase at the level of a stroke or cardiovascular injury from a heart attack. There is a direct relationship between low estrogen levels and increased rates of colon cancer in women. In patients suffering from chronic pain, estrogen has been shown to decrease pain sensitivity and impacts the pain pathways; it plays a vital role in building bone in both men and women, along with testosterone.

Estrogen decreases visceral fat, or fat around the vital organs. High levels of visceral fat are very inflammatory and highly linked to cardiovascular disease, metabolic syndrome, diabetes, and early death. Estrogen is also vital to brain health in both women and men. Research suggests that estrogen prevents Alzheimer's disease through its anti-inflammatory response, as well as decreasing what is called beta amyloid deposition, a hallmark of Alzheimer's disease. Estrogen has been shown to decrease cognitive decline, increase mental clarity and memory, and plays a very important role in moods and depression. The findings that have been reported over the past few decades have given great insight to the vital role estrogen plays in major chronic disease prevention.

WHERE DOES ESTROGEN ORIGINATE?

Estrogen in women is made from cholesterol by the ovaries and to a lesser extent from the adrenal gland via DHEA conversion. Estrogen is also made from an enzyme mentioned earlier called aromatase. Aromatase converts testosterone to estrogen in men in the exact ratios the body needs to be healthy. Some men may make less aromatase and do not get as high of estrogen conversion, and some men might make more aromatase than they need and have a higher estrogen conversion from testosterone. This is not necessarily a bad thing, as multiple studies have shown, a higher estrogen level in a male is correlated with prevention of cardiovascular disease, higher libido, and prevention of osteoporosis. Estrogen in men can also be created from DHEA, just like in females.

Sometimes, estrogen also gets a bad rap in males, but usually, that is in males who have high amounts of visceral fat. Estrogen is produced in adipose, or fat cells, via aromatase enzymes. There have been some poorly reported studies that have blamed estrogen for the increased rates of metabolic syndrome and cardiovascular disease in men with high levels of visceral fat. But what if the inflammatory visceral fat is actually the root cause? It can be very confusing when researching online,

"17β-estradiol (β=beta), the most potent estrogen in circulation, is shown to be anti-inflammatory and preventive of many chronic diseases, like heart disease, neurovascular disease, type 2 diabetes, hypertension, bone loss, and chronic pain syndromes in both women and men."

as you will likely find mixed information about estrogen in men. I always stick to what expert clinical studies show, that 17β-estradiol (β=beta), the most potent estrogen in circulation, is shown to be anti-inflammatory and preventive of many chronic diseases, like heart disease, neurovascular disease, type 2 diabetes, hypertension, bone loss, and chronic pain syndromes in both women and men.

Estrogen does its work by stimulating the estrogen receptors, which are present all over the body. Estrogen also easily crosses the "blood-brain barrier," which means it gets into the brain and stimulates the estrogen receptors that help with memory, moods, and thinking, and of course, prevention of all the diseases discussed earlier.

Are there some "bad estrogens" out there? You bet! These forms of estrogen are known as endocrine disruptors. I will talk more about endocrine disruptors later during the discussion of metabolism of estrogen, gut health, and certain supplements that can help positively impact estrogen metabolism.

ESTROGEN AND BREAST CANCER

Let's go ahead and get this conversation out of the way. A woman's biggest fear when it comes to discussing hormone replacement therapy is the unfounded fear of breast cancer. It may surprise you that estrogen therapy shows no risk in breast cancer survivors, and it does not increase breast cancer recurrence or mortality (dying from breast cancer). Estrogen is considered safe, even for breast cancer survivors! As I said previously, an incredible result of the WHI was published in the well-known medical journal JAMA in 2020. This long-term follow-up was reported on over 27,000 women over the course of 20 years. The authors reported that the estrogen-only arm of the trial showed that women on estrogen were significantly more protected against breast cancer and had significantly lower rates of breast cancer mortality (deaths) than women on no hormones. WOW! Now that flies in the face of everything the public has been told about estrogen for the past 20 years!

"Women on estrogen were significantly more protected against breast cancer and had significantly lower rates of breast cancer mortality (deaths) than women on no hormones."

So, now "they" are saying—wait, hold on, our mistake—estrogen, without synthetic progestin, actually protects women from breast cancer and death! Unfortunately, research has shown it takes medical providers on average 8-13 years to change their clinical practice after new information has been revealed about treating a certain disease process. At the time of this book writing, three years have passed since the JAMA article was published, and not one clinical guideline has changed; estrogen is still labeled in prescribing references as potentially cancer causing. Unless a healthcare provider stays up to date on this information, they are still prescribing based on outdated information, and tens of thousands of women are being denied a life altering medication.

Why has it taken so long for this information to come out? It truly boggles the mind!

There are hundreds of thousands of medical practitioners who have not read this long-term study and are still giving outdated advice to their patients, suggesting that they stay away from all hormone therapies to avoid risk of breast cancer. I observe this daily in my clinics. I hear it often from practitioners who come to the lectures and trainings I lead, and I have witnessed this in my own practice when patients choose to believe their primary care provider, discontinuing or never beginning their hormone optimization plan over unfounded fear of breast cancer. Sadly, many of these patients end up diagnosed with breast cancer a few years down the road because the root cause of the increased breast cancer risk- diet, nutritional deficiencies that aide in hormone metabolism, and other key issues - were not addressed.

Further, as it is not considered standard of care at the time this book was written, women with a history of breast cancer or have the BRCA gene, are told to avoid estrogen hormones at all costs, some even going so far as having their ovaries and breasts removed because the fear is so great and engrained (think Angelina Jolie). As you will see in the following sections, avoiding estrogen based on nonscientific recommendations may have dire consequences for your health.

For over a decade, I have researched and taught about the lack of evidence supporting estrogen's role in breast cancer causation or increased risk of death from breast cancer. I'm so grateful the clinical studies are finally reporting what the well-informed have known for 20 years. However, as it is still not standard of care to give an estrogen receptor positive breast cancer survivor estrogen hormone therapy, it is not recommended until the research catches up with the clinical practice guidelines and standards.

ESTROGEN AND BONES

It is a well-known and accepted fact that estrogen is critical for bone health. Research shows that women who avoid estrogen replacement therapy after menopause have a much higher risk of osteoporosis and osteoporotic fractures than women on estrogen, and when testosterone replacement is added to the regimen, bone building is even greater. It has been understood for decades that testosterone combined with estrogen has beneficial effects on bone building.

Two great studies from the late 80s and early 90s showed when testosterone therapy was added to estrogen, in a form described as continuous hormone therapy with hormone pellet implants, there was an additive effect on bone mineral density compared to using estrogen alone. That is because there is an abundance of estrogen and androgen receptors found on all three bone cells: osteoclasts, osteoblasts, and osteocytes, which illustrates the dual role in building bone. In the 1987 study on estrogen and testosterone pellet implants , not only did the results show a great increase in bone mineral density, but no adverse effects were observed either.

In the PEPI trial, an eight-year follow-up study on hormones and bone loss in postmenopausal women, results showed women who stopped using hormones, or never used hormones, had significant rates of bone loss compared to the women who stayed on their hormone therapy regimen.

The impact on continuous estrogen, progesterone, and testosterone replacement and bone has never been so evident as it was in the early days of treating patients with hormone pellet therapy. I had a patient who had been suffering from osteoporosis for almost a decade; nothing she tried, nor any medication she went on, improved her osteoporosis. After two years of continuous hormone replacement therapy with pellets, she excitedly brought the results of her most recent bone density test to my office. For the first time in more than a decade, she was building bone! Her osteoporosis had reversed to osteopenia. Fast forward another two years and her osteopenia had completely reversed, and her bone density scans were completely normal .

Estrogen is also a very important hormone for bone development in men. Testosterone and estrogen are critical for normal bone development, and as men age, they have a decline in both of these vital hormones. The age-related decrease in these hormones is associated with many health problems, including osteoporosis.

ESTROGEN AND THE HEART

For many years, I suffered from episodes of what is called supraventricular tachycardia. The condition began when I was about 18 years old, after having my first child, and continued with increasing frequency as I got older. This condition occurs when the heart starts beating very rapidly for no reason. It can be quite disconcerting, as the heart is beating so fast, blood is not pumping well to the brain, and on many occasions, I felt like I was going to pass out. I learned through the years in my clinical training there are certain maneuvers you can do to stop the erratic heartbeat, but there were two occasions I was unable to get it under control and was taken to the emergency room.

About a month before my last visit to the emergency room, I visited a cardiologist who specialized in arrhythmias. He told me I most likely needed to have what was called a cardiac ablation, where they find the pathway in your heart that is taking over the pacing and cauterize it so pathway stops working. It sounded extreme for something I was able to control my whole adult life and a possible side effect of the procedure was death, so I decided against it. That was, until the following week when I had another episode I could not stop. My neighbor took me to the local ER, and this time, the emergency room physician was not going to let me leave without treating me with a medication called adenosine.

I didn't like how it felt to have my heart stopped with this medication! That is what adenosine does; it literally stops your heart for a few seconds—feels like an eternity—and the hope is when your heart picks up beating again, it will be in a normal rhythm. The first injection, which felt exactly like heart attack has been described: a crushing painful sensation going down my left arm and traveling all the way down my left leg, didn't work. He ordered a second injection, ignoring my pleas to hold off and give it time. Thankfully, the second injection worked. I called my cardiologist from the hospital bed and scheduled an appointment for the ablation. The procedure was a success, and it would be another five or six years before I had issues with an irregular heartbeat again.

At the time, I hadn't recognized an interesting pattern; the episodes throughout the years coincided with my menstrual cycle. When I got into my late 40s and my menstrual cycles became more irregular due to perimenopause, I began to experience the same irregular heartbeat that previously led to the prolonged tachycardic episodes. I made another appointment with my cardiologist because I remembered him warning me the ablation might not last forever. I was afraid I was going to have to undergo the procedure again. I visited my cardiologist, and he put me on a cardiac monitor and did several tests but couldn't find anything amiss, so I decided to wait it out.

One day while I was preparing notes for a lecture on estrogen, it hit me like a ton of bricks: when estrogen is low or fluctuates, it can cause issues with the cardiac conduction, or put simply, your heartbeat. I decided to get my blood levels of estrogen checked, and sure enough, they were radically fluctuating due to perimenopause. I was immediately treated with a low dose of estrogen to level out the fluctuations. The erratic beating of my heart discontinued. Many of my patients have also experienced this issue when their estrogen gets low. I just couldn't see it in myself initially. Now, when I start having an irregular heartbeat, that's my signal that my estrogen is low, and it is time for my next hormone pellet therapy appointment. I will discuss hormone pellets later in the section on treatment options for hormone therapy.

Numerous studies throughout the decades have shown the positive impact estrogen has in the cardiovascular system. 17β-estradiol, the primary estrogen of the human body, has been shown to protect the heart from heart disease. Women who have transitioned through menopause and are on estrogen replacement therapy have been shown to have markedly reduced incidences of death from a heart attack.

" Numerous studies throughout the decades have shown the positive impact estrogen has in the cardiovascular system."

What about the statement that women should be on the lowest dose of hormone for the shortest amount of time possible or that women should not start hormone therapy after age 60? Well, that recommendation fell by the wayside in 2017, thank goodness. However, an interesting study, published in 2018 examined nearly 490,000 women on estrogen hormone therapy between 1994 and 2009. This study uncovered that not only was heart disease risk significantly reduced, but also the risk of stroke death and all causes of death were significantly reduced in women on menopausal hormone therapy. The study further stated all risk reductions were comparable in women who had started hormone therapy before 60 as well as women who started therapy after age 60. The old recommendation that you shouldn't start hormones after age 60 because of safety concerns has fallen out of favor. I wonder if your primary care provider knows that.

In the ELITE trial , the early-versus-late-intervention trial with estrogen, the authors wanted to examine the effects of oral estradiol on the progression of atherosclerosis in over 600 healthy post-menopausal women. The women in the study already had a subclinical (mild) atherosclerosis (a.k.a. "hardening of the arteries") present. What the authors found was women who started on estrogen early in the trial, on average within three years of menopause, showed a greater than 50 percent reduction in the rate of the progression of their heart disease compared to women not on estrogen therapy.

Not only is it safe for women of all ages, but some studies have shown it is dangerous for women to abruptly stop taking their estrogen. In two studies from 2016 and 2017, the authors noted estrogen had very important effects on the functioning of the heart, including blood pressure and endothelial relaxation, meaning the ability for the arteries to expand and contract, as well as development of enlargement of the heart, which leads to congestive heart failure. They noted discontinuation of estrogen is not recommended, as acute withdrawals from the circulation may predispose women to potentially fatal cardiovascular events! In a landmark 2016 study, the authors stated estrogen should be a preventive strategy not only for reducing bone loss and new onset of diabetes but also cardiovascular disease and all causes of death!

"Estrogen should be a preventive strategy not only for reducing bone loss and new onset of diabetes but also cardiovascular disease and all causes of death!"

What a bold statement! Drop the mic !

Estrogen has also been shown to have a positive impact in men and women's cholesterol levels. LDL, the so called "bad cholesterol", in women who were receiving estrogen pellet implants was decreased, and HDL was significantly increased. Another study showed that among men supplementing testosterone, the conversion to estrogen via aromatase decreased the total cholesterol and triglycerides and increased HDL cholesterol. An important study from 2007 in men showed estrogen is positively associated with apo-lipoprotein A, a beneficial cholesterol molecule, and regulation of blood pressure. When men had higher levels of estrogen, they showed a lower risk of cardiovascular disease.

When testosterone and estrogen are combined in hormone therapy regimens for women, added benefits to the cardiovascular system have been shown, including reductions in total cholesterol and LDL, reductions in belly fat, and increase in bone density and muscle mass. It's extremely important to optimize all your hormones, not just one. The human body was designed to work in harmony, and all the hormones are synergistic with one other, producing greater impact on health than just one hormone alone.

ESTROGEN AND THE BRAIN

An 82-year-old patient of mine has gone on and off hormones for almost a decade.

No matter how much I educated her, she just couldn't overcome her fear of estrogen. You see, she was told for many years by her primary care provider that estrogen would cause breast cancer. Over the past five years, she had noticed her memory becoming progressively worse. This really concerned her because in every other area of her life, she is very healthy and active! She was concerned that she was getting Alzheimer's disease and it caused her a great deal of anguish. The distress over her failing memory caused her to be depressed, and she didn't see the point in living. After much deliberation on her part, and after her son discussed extensively with her the unfounded fear of breast cancer, but the real danger of developing Alzheimer's disease, strokes, cardiovascular disease, and osteoporotic fractures, she reluctantly decided to go back on her hormones.

Within two weeks of being back on hormone therapy with estrogen, progesterone, and testosterone, her son and granddaughter reported she wasn't complaining about her memory, her moods were vastly improved and her depression and desire to die were gone.

Estrogen plays an incredibly important role in prevention of chronic disease processes that negatively impact the function of the brain. Estradiol has been shown to reduce the risk for Alzheimer's disease, cognitive decline, and memory loss. In a 2017 study on estrogen and Alzheimer's disease, when post-menopausal women on estrogen were compared to women not on estrogen for an average of 15 years, the women on estrogen experienced a marked increase in blood flow to the brain and a decreased risk of dementia. Further, the study showed estrogen protects the brain by decreasing beta amyloid, a protein that, when in great numbers, clusters together to form the plaques distinctive of Alzheimer's disease.

"Estrogen plays an incredibly important role in prevention of chronic disease processes that negatively impact the function of the brain."

The same study showed that progestins, not progesterone, can diminish the positive effects of estrogen on the brain and worsen Alzheimer's disease. That is contrary to the natural hormone progesterone, which has been shown to be synergistic to estrogen's positive role in the brain, much like testosterone. More on the differences between progesterone and progestins in a later chapter.

A landmark study published in early 2002 and updated in 2012 showed a 30 percent Alzheimer's reduction in women if they started estradiol hormone therapy within five years of menopause and when used for more than 10 years. Later research on this topic answers the question of "how" this happens. Estradiol, and estradiol via testosterone conversion, plays a key role in decreasing what is called beta-amyloid-induced apoptosis (cell death) by increasing the amount of a protein called BCL-xl. BCL-xl is a part of the BCL-2 family of proteins, which have been called the "anti-aging" proteins. They can help regulate healthy cell survival and unhealthy cell death, a process known as autophagy. Autophagy is a really cool thing the human body does naturally when all things at the cellular level are in harmony, in the medical field, this is termed as "homeostasis".

"Autophagy" is derived from the Greek autóphagos, meaning "self-devouring," and is a process naturally programmed in a cell that is not functioning properly. A function of aging, and the hormone decline that comes with aging, is insufficient autophagy. This may be a key reason why, as people age, the risk for several diseases that are a result of insufficient autophagy may increase.

Autophagy plays an important role as a tumor suppressor in cancer cases, and research has been underway looking for ways to increase targeted tumor cell death. Could it be that optimizing hormones to youthful levels, a time when age-related cancers are mostly nonexistent, seems a beneficial route to prevention?

What about strokes? Earlier in this book, I referenced the beneficial effects of estradiol on strokes and injury from strokes. Let's look at some research in this area. Research began in 2014 that was looking at the impact estradiol has on the brain following ischemic stroke. An ischemic stroke is usually caused by a clot, or plaque rupture, that stops blood flow to that area of the brain, and if not treated quickly, may cause that area of the brain to die. If an intervention is not made within minutes of the onset of the stroke, permanent brain death can occur, hence the devastating, and most often lifelong, consequences of disability following a stroke.

The researchers found at the level of a stroke injury, there is a large amount of estradiol created via the enzyme aromatase. This led them to believe estradiol must play a key role in protecting the brain after a stroke. Initial studies found estradiol activated several pathways that protected the brain, primarily through anti-inflammatory and immune response pathways. In a subsequent study, the researchers utilized 17β-estradiol in patients at a research hospital following a stroke and found that estradiol increased the amount of several proteins that were involved in cell survival. It also decreased certain proteins that were involved in cell death, called pro-apoptotic proteins. As an acute care practitioner who spent many years in emergency medicine and as a hospitalist taking care of stroke victims, this was very exciting news to me!

The most recent research on this area, published in 2023, agreed with the prior research that estrogens exert very important neuro-protective activities in the brain, and they have a profoundly positive impact on the immune system and inflammation, two areas known to be involved in strokes. The research emphasized that not only does estrogen protect against cell death but is vital for stimulation of new brain cells or neurons.

"Estrogens exert very important neuro-protective activities in the brain."

A key takeaway of the 2023 study emphasized the differences in the outcomes of estrogen on stroke and stroke progression *depend on the type of hormones used.* Progestins and synthetic estrogens, they stated, have profound and vastly different effects on the brain regarding prevention and protection when compared to 17β-estradiol and progesterone, the natural hormones made by the human body. This is why it is so important when you are researching replacing your hormones, you supplement with as close of a hormone molecule as our own body makes: 17β-estradiol, micronized progesterone and testosterone for women and testosterone for men.

ESTROGEN AND SKIN

The skin is the largest organ in the body. Yes, our skin is considered an organ! It's a living, breathing barrier between our insides and the outside world. It's often the first organ to show toxicity in the body, manifesting as acne, eczema, rosacea, and various rashes and bumps. Homeostasis (there's that word again) of the skin as a defensive barrier and conduit for good (and harmful) chemicals and substances is vitally important, and estrogen plays a key role in this organ's wellbeing.

Estrogen plays a significant role in not only cosmetic appearance of skin—think fine lines, wrinkles, dry and crepey skin, and "age spots" — but also in wound healing and immune responses. An immunomodulator is a substance that modifies the immune response to help the body fight disease or illness. Remember in the previous section about the heart and the brain how estrogen functions as an anti-inflammatory agent and an immunomodulator? Well, the same processes are happening in the skin, much like the brain, heart, and many other organs or systems in the body. Estrogen increases collagen and elasticity in the skin, as well as thickness, and besides keeping us looking youthful, that firm thicker skin keeps us warm too.

There are estrogen receptors in every layer of the skin, also called the dermal layers, indicating the role estrogen plays not only in the cosmetic appearances of our skin, but also hair growth, sweat and oil gland function, which keep our skin hydrated and dewy in appearance. The thinning that occurs after menopause without estrogen replacement matches the same rate of bone loss in women who don't replace their estrogen after menopause. The collagen content in the skin decreases by 30 percent in the early menopause years and then at a rate of 2 percent per year after menopause.

"The collagen content in the skin decreases by 30 percent in the early menopause years and then at a rate of 2 percent per year after menopause."

The age-related changes that occur with menopause can be largely reversed with replacing natural estrogen, but like all the other body processes discussed up until now, the benefits are enhanced when you replace all the hormones that are deficient: estrogen, testosterone, and progesterone in women and testosterone, which converts to estrogen naturally, in men. Clinical observations of patients on hormone replacement therapy with 17β-estradiol show improvements in skin thickness, hydration, wrinkles, and elasticity, as well as reversing the altered wound healing and inflammation that happens when hormones begin to decline.

As I wrap up the conversation about estrogen, I must emphasize how vitally important this hormone is. Before I transitioned through menopause, I didn't give estrogen as much credit as testosterone for helping patients feel better. What I came to realize, is estrogen is vitally important. When my estrogen is low, my brain is tired. I have had women state this for years - now I know the difference: low estrogen causes a brain fatigue; low testosterone causes a body fatigue. When estrogen levels are restored to youthful ranges, skin elasticity and dewiness is improved, belly fat decreases, the brain works better, moods are better, everything is just better!

CHAPTER 4

PROGESTERONE

Progesterone, named from the root words "pro" and "gestation," meaning for pregnancy, is a very important hormone for women. At one time, it was believed progesterone was only beneficial for the premenopausal female to regulate menstrual cycles and maintain pregnancy. It is now known there are progesterone receptors in many of the same areas of the body as estrogen and testosterone, indicating the important role they all play in many body systems. The brain, bone, breast tissue, and reproductive organs in females all rely heavily on the influence of progesterone on the progesterone receptors. Progesterone receptors have been identified in many body systems and are activated in a variety of functions.

Progesterone opposes estrogen's influence in some areas of the body, like the uterus and the breasts, and balances the effect of estrogen during premenstrual syndrome when women experience more fluid retention, bloating, and headaches. As one colleague has put it, "progesterone is key to life," as life cannot begin without adequate progesterone, and life can come to an end due to a lack of progesterone, look at its impact on rates of colon cancer, endometrial, ovarian, skin, and prostate cancers.

Progesterone is synthesized in the brain and is considered a "neurosteroid" like estrogen and testosterone. It is a key player in new brain cell and neuron development, impacts learning and mood, and has been successfully used in clinical trials as an infusion after a traumatic brain injury, reducing brain swelling and improving recovery. This hormone has also been shown to protect the brain after stroke, alongside estrogen and independently of estrogen and has been shown to be beneficial in Alzheimer's disease, as it plays a key role in inflammation and immune response. Decline of progesterone is also a primary root cause of post-partum depression.

Decline of progesterone is also a primary root cause of post-partum depression.

One of my mentors whom I've learned a great deal from in the hormone space, Dr. Neal Rouzier, is incredibly passionate about progesterone. He is an emergency room physician by training who, over the course of the years, learned about the benefits of hormone optimization, started a clinic, and has been teaching in this space all over the world for over three decades. When he teaches about progesterone, he tells a story about a woman who came into the emergency room one evening complaining of depression.

He described it as a very busy evening in the emergency room, and apparently, the nursing staff was quite perturbed that this seemingly well put-together executive female would waste everyone's time coming to the emergency room with this complaint. After they got her to a room, several hours passed, and when Dr. Rouzier was finally able to see her, he asked the usual questions regarding what brought her into the emergency department. The patient shared that she had a baby about six weeks prior, and she felt like she wanted to kill her baby and then kill herself; she didn't have a plan. She was just very scared.

In that moment, Dr. Rouzier was quite certain he knew exactly what she needed and ordered a shot of 400 mg progesterone to be administered. He told her, "I'm going to come back and check on you in an hour." When he checked back in, she looked like a completely different person, and she asked him, "What did you give me? I can't believe how much better I feel." He went on to explain how after having a baby, progesterone levels can be very low and take some time to come back up. She was simply very deficient in progesterone and needed some help while her body got back in order. He put her on a prescription for oral progesterone every night at a higher dose than usual and told her to follow up with her gynecologist in a few weeks and have her levels checked.

"Progesterone has been referred to as a "calming hormone."

Progesterone has been referred to as a "calming hormone," and when taken the week before the menstrual cycle, can greatly decrease the bloating and effects of premenstrual syndrome. Taken at night, it aids in a restful sleep and taken as a dissolvable tablet under the tongue during the day, it may decrease anxiety. Several of my colleagues who treat teenage girls have used it quite successfully, in much lower doses, to address mood swings and anxiety related to the hormone changes that accompany puberty.

The mother of a 13-year-old patient of one of my colleagues was so desperate for some help with her daughter she was willing to try anything! Her daughter's moods and erratic behavior were disrupting the household, and she was waking up at night with anxiety attacks; the practitioner placed her on a low dose of oral progesterone at night and completely stopped all those problems.

The benefits of progesterone on mood and anxiety are thought to derive from progesterone stimulation of the GABA system, as well as its impact on serotonin levels in the brain. Neurotransmitters are chemical messengers, like hormones, that transmit messages in the nervous system. GABA is a brain neurotransmitter that balances excitability in the brain, it is calming. It has been shown in many cases to be more effective than antidepressants, most notably when mood disorders are related to hormone fluctuations. Serotonin is a neurotransmitter that helps to regulate mood, appetite, sleep and sexual function and causes feelings of happiness, contentment and relaxation.

Progesterone has also been successfully used to treat menstrual-related migraines, and the time of life when a woman begins to have very heavy cycles that are closer together, usually starting in the early 40s, taking progesterone at night can regulate and lighten those heavy cycles. This is because at about age 40, progesterone levels begin to decline, and low progesterone with normal estrogen levels causes the lining of the uterus to grow, which results in what is called "dysfunctional uterine bleeding."

It is important to understand there is a big difference between natural progesterone, also known as bioidentical progesterone or micronized progesterone, and the synthetic form of progesterone called progestin. Progestins vastly differ from natural progesterone, from the receptors they target to the actions on the cells and the side effects—all are completely opposite of natural progesterone. For example, synthetic progestins are known to cause extreme birth defects in a developing baby; however, natural progesterone is vital to maintain a pregnancy in the first trimester. Without enough progesterone, the pregnant woman will suffer a miscarriage (hence the root meaning of the name). Progesterone has been shown to protect the breasts against breast cancer, but progestins are the only hormone class that have been shown in any clinical study to increase the risk of breast cancer. Progestins also increase breast pain and swelling; however, progesterone decreases these effects. Synthetic progestins also have significant side effects like depression, anxiety, fatigue, headaches, increased blood clots, water retention, and lowering of our "good" HDL cholesterol - all opposite of natural progesterone!

Although the adrenal glands and testes produce a very low amount of progesterone in males, the hormone has not been shown to be clinically useful in treating hormone decline in men. Progesterone seems to be related to the production of sperm, but beyond that function, it has not been widely studied as a vital hormone for men. The limited research on progesterone use in men is related to using it for specific non-hormonal issues, such as brain trauma, cardiovascular issues, COVID recovery, smoking cessation, and other drug withdrawal treatments.

To recap, progesterone is a hormone that plays a crucial role in various physiological processes in both males and females. Some of the benefits of progesterone include:

1. **Regulating the menstrual cycle:** Progesterone is involved in the regulation of the menstrual cycle in women. It helps prepare the uterus for pregnancy by thickening the uterine lining (endometrium) and maintaining its integrity. In cases of hormonal imbalance, progesterone supplementation can help regulate the menstrual cycle.

2. **Supporting pregnancy**: Progesterone is often referred to as the "pregnancy hormone" as it is vital for maintaining a healthy pregnancy. It helps to sustain the uterine lining, prevents contractions that could lead to premature labor, and supports fetal development.

3. **Reducing symptoms of premenstrual syndrome (PMS):** Progesterone can alleviate symptoms associated with PMS, such as bloating, breast tenderness, mood swings, and irritability. It helps balance hormone levels and can provide relief for women experiencing severe PMS symptoms.

4. **Supporting bone health:** Progesterone plays a role in maintaining bone density. It aids in the deposition of new bone tissue and helps prevent bone loss, especially during menopause when estrogen levels decline. Progesterone therapy may be beneficial in preventing osteoporosis and reducing the risk of fractures.

5. **Supporting cardiovascular health:** Progesterone has been shown to have positive effects on cardiovascular health. It helps to regulate blood pressure, reduce

inflammation, and improve lipid profiles, which can contribute to a lower risk of cardiovascular disease.

6. **Enhancing mood and promoting relaxation:** Progesterone has a calming effect on the central nervous system. It can help improve mood, reduce anxiety, and promote a sense of relaxation and well-being.

7. **Supporting brain function:** Progesterone receptors are present in the brain, and progesterone is involved in various neurological processes. It may enhance cognitive function, memory, and protect against neurodegenerative diseases.

8. **Supporting healthy skin:** Progesterone plays a role in maintaining healthy skin by promoting collagen production and reducing skin dryness. It can help improve skin elasticity and reduce the appearance of wrinkles.

CHAPTER 5

TESTOSTERONE

"Testosterone is so important for a sense of well-being when you get older."
Sylvester Stallone

Sly Stallone's comment about sense of well-being cannot be overstated! I have heard countless patients share the same sentiment, men, and women alike. Testosterone is the feel-good hormone. When it is low or sub optimal (left side of the reference range) a myriad of vague symptoms are present. Things like fatigue, especially in the afternoon between two and four pm, brain fog, short term memory loss- like "why did I come in this room? Where did I park my car"? Irritability and moodiness, anxiety, insomnia, waking up between two and four in the morning - these are just some of the symptoms low testosterone can cause. And of course, a lack of sex drive for women and, although the last symptom to present in men, erectile dysfunction.

Compounded, these daily issues can wreak havoc on relationships - marriages most notably. I have had countless relationships restored after one or both partners optimized their hormones.

It reminds me of a young male patient who retired early from the military as a paratrooper because of debilitating depression and fatigue, erratic mood swings and extreme anger episodes. His wife became the primary breadwinner while he endlessly sought help and treatment for his symptoms. His doctors at the military clinic could not seem to find an answer. He continued to gain weight, which worsened his depression and self-worth. He became a nightmare to live with, his wife and children tiptoed around him, and the household was constantly tense. His wife heard about our clinics and when doing research realized her husband had all the symptoms described that were related to low testosterone, so she made him an appointment.

After evaluating his blood work and his history, he had several concussions from his job, he was found not only to have very low, double digits low, testosterone, but also severe leaky gut syndrome. This makes sense as repeated head injuries and concussions, whether mild or severe, profoundly impact the pituitary gland where luteinizing hormone is secreted that stimulates testicular production of testosterone. Moreover, within about 30 minutes of a head injury, intestinal permeability, or leaky gut, can occur. More on leaky gut later.

We began treating him with testosterone, addressed nutritional, gut, and other deficiencies and for the first time in 4 years, both husband and wife felt some hope for the future. When I saw him again the following month, he was a completely different person. I almost didn't recognize him; he couldn't believe the changes either. He tried to tell his military doctors about his treatment and tried to continue his treatment through the military clinic for cost reasons, but sadly it fell on deaf ears.

Testosterone is the most abundant active hormone in men and women. This may surprise you, but yes, women make and need testosterone. It is a vital hormone for everyone across their lifespan. There are receptors for testosterone in every single body system: the hair follicle, skin, and scalp; the brain, spinal cord, nerve tissue, eyes, and ears; the thyroid and other endocrine glands; cardiovascular tissue, breast tissue, lung tissue; the uterus and vagina, the G.I. tract, muscles, bone and fat cells. Head to toe, testosterone impacts more body systems than any other sex hormone.

"Testosterone is the most abundant active hormone in men and women."

"Head to toe, testosterone impacts more body systems than any other sex hormone."

Testosterone is primarily produced in the testes in males and in smaller amounts in the ovaries and adrenal glands in females. Specialized cells called Leydig cells, located within the testes, produce and release testosterone in response to signals from the luteinizing hormone (LH) secreted by the pituitary gland. This process is known as testicular or Leydig cell testosterone production. The ovaries in females produce testosterone, although in much smaller quantities compared to males. The ovarian production of testosterone occurs in the ovarian stromal cells and is regulated by luteinizing hormone (LH) and follicle-stimulating hormone (FSH). The adrenal glands, located above the kidneys, also contribute to the production of testosterone. The adrenal cortex, specifically the zona reticularis, produces and releases testosterone as well as other androgens.

Testosterone has been shown in many clinical studies to aid in the prevention and even treatment of many chronic disease processes: heart disease, Alzheimer's disease, depression and other mood disorders, breast cancer, prostate cancer, memory and cognitive decline, diabetes and insulin resistance, chronic and acute pain syndromes, and osteoporosis; the list goes on and on. Let's deep dive into a few of these areas.

TESTOSTERONE AND THE HEART

All the systems, organs, and cells in our body depend on our blood supply, and our blood supply is directly dependent on what is called the endothelial cells. Endothelial cells are a rich network of life in and of themselves, and the work they do is vital to supporting life: the endothelial cells line the entire vascular system. "What does this have to do with testosterone?" you may ask. Well, in a nutshell, everything!

Testosterone has been shown in several studies to be beneficial for endothelial cells, as testosterone induces what is called nitric oxide production, which is vital for the regeneration, motility (or movement), and growth of endothelial cells. Testosterone also blocks inflammation and stickiness of endothelial cells, as well as decreases clotting, demonstrating "anti-thrombotic" (anti-clotting) properties.

Testosterone has been shown in many studies to be highly beneficial to the heart and the cardiovascular system, owing much to the influence on the endothelial lining. Low blood levels of testosterone in men and women have been shown to increase the risk of many diseases related to the heart, like elevated cholesterol, adverse blood clotting, being overweight, and insulin resistance, all of which lead to type 2 diabetes. Low testosterone, or "low T," is also associated with higher cortisol levels, increased belly fat, and atherosclerosis or "hardening of the arteries." Low T is correlated with higher total cholesterol, high LDL cholesterol, high triglycerides, increased inflammation, and increased thickness of the artery walls, which contributes to the endothelial lining to becoming dysfunctional.

It is important to understand the relationship between inflammation and chronic diseases. Heart disease is not a disease caused by excess cholesterol as once believed. Cholesterol is necessary in the correct amounts, types, and ratios for many processes in the body, not the least of which is hormone production. But when testosterone is low, or "low-normal," the body increases the amounts and activity of a substance called NF-kappa B, which causes the overproduction of what is called inflammatory cytokines and other immune factors. These inflammatory and immune factors go into overdrive, and the chronic inflammation that results alters endothelial function, which leads to high blood pressure. High blood pressure leads to more stress on the heart and thus more stress on the body because it decreases blood flow to vital organs, which increases inflammation, and the cycle just continues.

In men, blood testosterone levels are inversely related to all causes of death, including death from cardiovascular disease. What that means is the lower the testosterone level, the higher the risk of all causes of death. In one study of over

11,000 men, the researchers showed the lower the testosterone in men, the higher rates of death from all causes, and they further related those deaths to endothelial dysfunction. I am going to talk a bit more later about what "normal" testosterone levels are. The same issues hold true for women. In one study that specifically looked at testosterone levels in post-menopausal women who had severe heart disease, they found, like their male counterparts, the inverse relationship between low testosterone levels and heart disease held true. What they concluded was the post-menopausal women who had higher levels of testosterone were protected against the development, and worsening, of heart disease.

Type 2 diabetes, sometimes referred to as adult-onset diabetes, although no longer exclusive to adults, is a preventable and reversible chronic disease. This is different than type 1 diabetes, where the pancreas stops producing insulin. Type 2 diabetes is associated with insulin resistance and inflammation from higher levels of visceral fat, or the fat that accumulates around the organs of the belly. Low testosterone is associated with worsening heart disease risk in people with type 2 diabetes and is also associated with insulin resistance and type 2 diabetes. This makes sense again when you understand the underlying cause: *inflammation.*

Which came first? Inflammation, belly fat, insulin resistance, and then diminished testosterone production or vice versa? I personally believe it's the former: inflammation increasing belly fat from a Western diet of processed foods and seed oils. More on this topic later when we discuss dietary influences of hormone production and metabolism.

TESTOSTERONE AND THE BRAIN

Mr. Jacks is the 93-year-old father of one of my patients who, just a few years prior to his initial visit with me, was a vigorous, active, mentally sharp man who lived on his own quite successfully. His daughter, Joanie, noticed her father becoming less and less active, choosing to stay in his recliner all day rather than get up for his morning walks and crossword puzzle games. The progression from active to sedentary was so slow and progressive she didn't notice much until one day, she went to visit him, and he kept saying he just felt so tired and washed out; he didn't want to get up out of bed.

She called his doctor for an appointment but couldn't be seen until the following week. She called me to ask my opinion, as she didn't want to wait a week for answers. His gradual symptoms did not seem urgent, and after I ran through worst-case scenarios and ruled them out, I urged her to have his doctor check his testosterone levels, along with the other blood and urine tests. She called me about three weeks later with his results: his blood level of testosterone was an 8! Critically low by anyone's standards! All his other tests came back negative as a source for his symptoms. At the urging and insistence of Joanie, his doctor reluctantly put him on a low dose of testosterone via a weekly injection. Joanie couldn't believe the change in him over the next few weeks. She told me it was like watching a dead person slowly come back to life; every day, he became brighter and brighter and more like his old self. By day five after his first shot, he was up, getting his shoes on to go for a walk. Remember the Greek

"It was like watching a dead person slowly come back to life."

meaning for the word "hormone," "arouse to activity"? It was never so visually evident as in the story of Mr. Jacks.

Testosterone is a powerful brain hormone. There are thousands of receptors for testosterone in the areas of our brain that are responsible for mood, thinking, mental clarity and focus. Low levels of testosterone in men and women are associated with depression, anxiety, mood swings, and cognitive impairment, such as memory loss and difficulty focusing. It is a fundamental hormone for psychological health in both males and females.

"Low levels of testosterone in men and women are associated with depression, anxiety, mood swings, and cognitive impairment, such as memory loss and difficulty focusing."

Testosterone can control the activity of neurotransmitters in the brain, such as acetylcholine, dopamine, and serotonin, which are involved in cognitive processes and mood regulation. Physical and mental stamina are also closely linked to testosterone production and decline in levels profoundly impacts energy levels and vigor.

Depression and low testosterone were the focus of my doctoral research in 2016 when I noticed after several years of prescribing testosterone therapy to women, many of them were able to successfully come off their antidepressant medication. I thought, this isn't a coincidence, so I began to study it at a deeper level. Lo and behold, I found in clinical research, there is a direct correlation between testosterone and depression.

All three sex hormones, testosterone, estrogen, and progesterone, influence depression greatly in women, but testosterone plays a key role in mental health across the lifespan of a female. Women who transition through menopause will experience worsening of their depression and anxiety because of the fluctuating levels of estrogen and the drop in progesterone levels. Within 24 hours of women undergoing a full hysterectomy, removal of both the uterus and the ovaries, testosterone levels drop by over 70 percent. Women who are on birth control pills will have low testosterone for two reasons: first and foremost, birth control pills stop the ovarian production of sex hormones and raise levels of a protein called sex hormone-binding globulin, which binds up free testosterone, worsening the already low testosterone levels.

Estrogen and testosterone also play a role in serotonin levels, and when these hormones are deficient, serotonin levels become altered and exacerbate the depressive symptoms of low testosterone. The good news is, in both women and men, testosterone replacement therapy can completely reverse the symptoms of depression when associated with hormone decline.

Women who are diagnosed with postpartum depression often have a testosterone and/or progesterone deficiency. Many of my female patients would complain after their second baby that they never felt the same; they never bounced back with their energy levels or libido, and their moods were awful. There is a direct correlation between childbearing and testosterone decline. This does not bode well for a healthy relationship with husbands, children, or anyone for that matter!

Further, as a woman progresses into her fourth decade of life, testosterone levels, along with progesterone levels, continue to fall rapidly. By the time a female is in her fifth decade of life, her testosterone levels have decreased even further, worsening an already compromised sense of well-being.

Testosterone levels can begin to decline in women any time across the lifespan, from childbearing years well into post-menopause, and for men, decline typically starts in their 30s and accelerates as men get into their fourth and fifth decades of life.

Unfortunately, cases of younger and younger people with lower testosterone levels are occurring at a rapid rate. This is because of what is known as endocrine disruptors. More on endocrine disruptors later when I talk about nutrition and nutritional influences on hormone production and metabolism.

Testosterone, like estrogen, also plays a role in prevention of Alzheimer's disease. Testosterone has neuroprotective actions, meaning it protects the neurological system from breakdown and progression into chronic diseases like Alzheimer's and age-related cognitive decline. Testosterone may have a direct neuroprotective effect on brain cells. It has been observed to promote neuronal survival, strengthen, and protect against cell damage and apoptosis (programmed cell death). These effects may help preserve brain function and prevent the degeneration of brain cells that is characteristic of Alzheimer's disease.

Testosterone also has anti-inflammatory properties, which can be beneficial in the context of Alzheimer's disease. Chronic inflammation in the brain is thought to contribute to the development and progression of Alzheimer's, and testosterone may help reduce this inflammation, potentially slowing down the disease process. Further, as discussed in the estrogen section, beta-amyloid plaques are abnormal protein aggregates that accumulate in the brains of individuals with Alzheimer's disease. Testosterone has been found to influence the production and clearance of beta-amyloid plaques, reducing their accumulation and associated neurotoxicity.

"Chronic inflammation in the brain is thought to contribute to the development and progression of Alzheimer's, and testosterone may help reduce this inflammation, potentially slowing down the disease process."

TESTOSTERONE AND THE BONES

Clinical studies date back for decades showing the relationship between the sex hormones and bone development, and since the 1980s, the addition of testosterone to a woman's hormone therapy regimen has been shown to exponentially increase bone density and decrease osteoporosis rates. Several studies in males show there is a direct correlation between testosterone decline and osteoporosis rates as well.

In one clinical study of postmenopausal women, the researchers compared the bone density rates with testosterone alone versus testosterone with estrogen and compared different modalities of hormone replacement, such as testosterone pellets against creams, patches, and oral therapies. What the researchers found was overwhelmingly significant: subcutaneous pellets increased bone building by greater than 6 percent over the other modalities. When thinking about it logically, it is most likely not only because of the synergistic effect between testosterone and estrogen with bone turnover and bone building, but also the fact that hormone pellets keep your levels elevated 24/7 for about 3-5 months, rather than having brief increases in levels over the course of hours or days with the other modalities.

"When the treatment closely mimics the natural structure, levels, production, and release of hormones, the better the outcomes."

The same theory holds true for all the long-term benefits observed in my clinics with hormone pellet therapy. When the treatment closely mimics the natural structure, levels, production, and release of hormones, the better the outcomes. Of course, no one can exactly replicate the perfection of how the human body is designed from birth into young adulthood, but I believe subcutaneous pellet therapy is as close as humanly possible to how God designed our bodies to function.

TESTOSTERONE AND THE BREASTS

Sandi is a 55-year-old patient of mine who had been on hormone therapy for many years when she was diagnosed with low-grade breast cancer in her right breast. The cancer was caught early, and she was able to have it removed. There was no lymph node involvement. She underwent radiation treatment, and her oncologist placed her on a drug called tamoxifen to block her estrogen receptors from any estrogen her body may still be producing, even though she was seven years post-menopausal. I hadn't seen Sandi in a while, and I knew it was because her oncologist refused to let her continue testosterone therapy because he, like many oncologists, was not educated on the powerful influence that testosterone has on protecting the breast against breast cancer. He was also not aware of the clinical studies that utilized testosterone to reverse breast cancer. After about nine months on tamoxifen, Sandi had spoken to her primary care provider about what she was experiencing and what her best options were; she was miserable.

He informed her, much to my pleasant surprise, that if she stayed off hormones and on the estrogen receptor blocker, there was no proof in research that it would prevent a recurrence of breast cancer. And to make matters worse, she was at greater risk of developing heart disease, Alzheimer's disease, strokes, or osteoporosis—just to name a few. She fell into depression because of the weight gained during her treatment along with her disinterest in sex with her husband because intercourse had become painful. Her depression and moodiness seemed to worsen every day. She took her primary care doctor's advice and made a visit to see me again. A year later, back on therapy, she is looking and feeling like her old self again.

I believe this is one of the most overlooked and underdeveloped conversations regarding breast cancer, the relationship between testosterone deficiency and breast cancer rates and the relationship between testosterone treatment and protection against breast cancer. Remember when I talked about the word "homeostasis" in a prior chapter? Breast homeostasis is one of the most important conversations in the hormone world and no one is talking about it.

"Breast homeostasis is one of the most important conversations in the hormone world and no one is talking about it."

Historically, conversations around hormones and breast cancer are best summed up in the proverbial statement "throwing the baby out with the bathwater." Practitioners and the public at large have been led to believe that hormones cause an increased risk of breast cancer. Well, if that was the case, then why don't more young women have higher rates of breast cancer when their hormone levels are at their peak? Estrogen and progesterone levels are extremely high during pregnancy, but increased rates of breast cancer in pregnant women are not seen. This begs the question of what is the correlation between aging and increased breast cancer risk? Well, there are many things that impact breast cancer risk: lifestyle and dietary factors notwithstanding, endocrine disruptors, family history, and genetic predispositions that don't cause breast cancer but can increase the risk when other factors altering breast homeostasis are present, are all considerations.

The breasts are rich with androgen (a.k.a. testosterone) receptors, and when the ratio between stimulatory estrogens and the protective androgens are out of balance, breast homeostasis is impacted. Testosterone has been shown in clinical studies to have an inhibitory and an anti-growth effect on breast tissue, balancing the stimulatory effect of estrogen on breast tissue. Multiple large-scale studies on testosterone used in women, primarily hormone pellets, have shown a statistically significant reduction in breast cancer rates among women who are on continuous testosterone replacement compared to women who are not.

Further, in the 1960s, some incredible research was reported that has been buried in old medical journals for the past 60 years. In these early studies, researchers studied women who had metastatic, end-of-life breast cancer. These women had endured the conventional treatments of breast cancer at the time and could not be cured. They placed the women on injectable testosterone at relatively high doses every two weeks and continued therapy until the disease reversed, slowed down, or the patient passed away. What they uncovered was that the metastatic cancer regressed, or reversed, in 17 percent of the women and stabilized in 42 percent of the women.

Dr. Rebecca Glazier, a breast cancer surgeon whose research primarily focuses on testosterone therapy in women, wrote a case study about a woman in her 70s who was diagnosed with a breast tumor and resisted the traditional routes of breast cancer treatment. Dr. Glazier utilized testosterone pellets that also had a substance in them called anastrozole, which decreases the conversion of testosterone to estrogen, and placed these pellets around the tumor in the patient's fatty tissue of the breast. The results were astounding. Within 13 weeks, the tumor volume had decreased 12-fold, and by 19 weeks, the tumor had reduced to a fraction of its original size! In 2019, she published a paper that compiled much of her life's work up to that moment. She stated that not only is testosterone protective to the breast but also should be investigated as a preventive strategy for breast cancer. When she put her data into an algorithm that predicts the average breast cancer rates in the general population and compared them to the population of her patients, breast cancer incidences were reduced by almost 50

"Not only is testosterone protective to the breast but also should be investigated as a preventive strategy for breast cancer."

percent in the women who were on continuous testosterone therapy with pellets.

In another similar study on continuous testosterone replacement with pellet therapy, the authors published results from 10 years' worth of data that showed not only were their breast cancer rates similar to Dr. Glazier's outcomes but significantly less than the rates shown in other studies that looked at breast cancer in the general population, including the Women's Health Initiatives, and the Million Women Study. The difference in this author's patient database compared to Dr. Glazier's was that some also received estrogen and testosterone in their treatment plan. What they found in both groups—the estrogen plus testosterone or testosterone-only group—had breast cancer rates that were significantly lower than prior studies of the general population. They concluded that testosterone alone and testosterone with estrogen hormone pellets did not increase the rate of breast cancer but, in fact, significantly reduced breast cancer incidence.

Anecdotally, in my own clinical practice across tens of thousands of hormone pellet procedures on females, our breast cancer rates coincide with the previously referenced data. This begs the question, why isn't this vital hormone being studied more for protection and prevention against breast cancer?

In this country, every October, for decades, companies, sports teams, and individuals proudly wear a pink ribbon and donate millions of dollars toward breast cancer research and finding the cure. However, a "cure" seems to be staring us right in the face in the form of prevention. A wise doctor once told me the best way to cure cancer is to never get it! Prevention is key.

Don't mishear me; I am not saying testosterone is the end-all, be-all "cure", but it certainly is interesting when you look at the facts surrounding this amazing hormone. When combined with other research assessing causes of cancer in general - obesity, smoking, sedentary lifestyle, dietary intake of sugar- are all factors and these same factors lead to issues with hormone metabolism. Upon closer examination of the body as a whole and not just one area, there are likely simple answers to these complex questions.

"When combined with other research assessing causes of cancer in general- obesity, smoking, sedentary lifestyle, dietary intake of sugar- are all factors and these same factors lead to issues with hormone metabolism."

Something to consider, and this is just my opinion based on researching this area for almost 15 years, simple things like diet, exercise, and lifestyle factors, plus adequate, quality hormone replacement therapy that induces whole-body homeostasis, isn't really a very sexy approach. Sadly, I don't think anyone is going to win the Nobel Prize for a cure to breast cancer with these basic theories. What's more, changing diet and lifestyle, looking at nutritional factors, and optimizing hormones and hormone metabolism is not a very lucrative answer to the breast cancer "cure".

TESTOSTERONE AND THE PROSTATE

Now let's talk about prostate cancer. I will say that the development in this area for men is much more advanced than the conversation about breast cancer and women.

There is, however, still a great deal of misinformation about testosterone in men as it relates to prostate cancer. Let's just start with one very important study that looked at testosterone receptors in the prostate. Dr. Abraham Morgentaler, like his counterpart in the testosterone and breast cancer arena Dr. Rebecca Glazier, is a pioneer in the area of testosterone and prostate cancer.

In 2012, Dr. Morgentaler published a paper that examined what is now referred to as the saturation model of the prostate. He discovered that there are a finite number of testosterone receptors in the prostate, and any testosterone level greater than 240 was not able to stimulate the prostate tissue. This is such important news because so many males who are diagnosed with prostate cancer have levels that are well above 240, yet not only are they denied testosterone therapy but also may be treated with testosterone blockers and hormone disruptors such as Casodex and Lupron and, in some cases, be castrated to stop testosterone production! These drugs and castration procedure completely drop testosterone levels to zero, creating side effects and misery for male patients, many of whom have told me is worse than the possibility of dying from prostate cancer.

Further, Dr. Morgentaler reports that there is no credible evidence to support this generalized theory that higher testosterone levels are dangerous, and low testosterone levels are somehow protective against prostate cancer. There is not any clinical evidence to support that the testosterone lowering drugs or castration prolong the life of prostate cancer survivors, certainly not with any quality. In fact, more and more evidence is showing that depriving a male of his vital hormones may slow the growth of a prostate cancer but also exponentially increases his rates of cardiovascular disease, insulin resistance and type 2 diabetes, risk for Alzheimer's disease, stroke, and osteoporosis. Not to mention pain, erectile dysfunction, depression, and the impaired quality of life that affects all his relationships, not the least of which with his spouse.

"Low testosterone is predictive of prostate cancer risk and risk of death from prostate cancer."

What is incredibly important for males, their family members, and their doctors to understand is low testosterone is predictive of prostate cancer risk and risk of death from prostate cancer. In one paper, the authors looked at 197 studies of men on testosterone therapy and found testosterone administration did not increase the risk of prostate cancer, and increased blood levels of androgens were not related to the risk of developing prostate cancer. In another study, males were treated with testosterone after one year of being treated for prostate cancer, and when normal prostate-specific antigen (PSA) was restored, there was zero-increased risk of recurrence rate of prostate cancer. The PSA is a blood test that screens for prostate specific antigens, that when elevated, suggest there is something going on with the prostate. Elevations do not mean you have prostate cancer but can be an early sign that something should be investigated.

The takeaway message from multiple studies regarding testosterone and prostate cancer is this: men with high testosterone are not at risk, low testosterone is not protective but is actually predictive of prostate cancer, low testosterone is associated with higher grade prostate cancer and a later stage diagnosis. Once a man has undergone treatment and his PSA is back to normal, it is safe to resume testosterone replacement therapy.

TESTOSTERONE AND PAIN

Alice is a 53-year-old woman who heard me speak during a hormone webinar. She was referred to the event by a colleague who is one of my patients. Unbeknownst to Alice, her staff had growing concerns about her loss of memory, forgetting things she had said in prior meetings, forgetting commitments, and her tendency to fly off the handle at small things that would not have affected her that way a decade prior. Even though her staff urged her to get things checked out, and my patient who worked for her urged her to see me for hormones, the advice went unheeded until I was invited to speak at a webinar hosted by a colleague in her network. After she heard me talk about the benefits of hormones in all the areas mentioned so far in this book: moods, memory, energy, stamina, sleep, disease prevention, and so forth, she began to pay attention when I spoke about pain. Denial is powerful. Alice had suffered from extreme foot pain every morning for the prior several years.

She didn't understand why it was happening, but gradually, as the morning wore on, the pain dissipated, and she soon forgot about it—an out-of-sight, out-of-mind sort of thing. She decided to see me as a patient to get her hormones checked as the root cause of her daily pain. After a consultation and evaluation of her bloodwork and history, she decided to move forward with hormone treatment. Two weeks later, she called, cautiously optimistic, stating that when she awoke that morning, her foot pain was gone. She couldn't believe it and was afraid it was temporary or some sort of placebo effect. I assured her it likely was not and reminded her of all the ways estrogen and testosterone impact pain and pain processing. Fast forward three months later to our next visit, the pain was still gone, and she was "hooked" (her term) on the increased energy and focus she noticed while on the hormones. Now, a patient for life, she continues to refer people from her network all over the world to me or a practitioner in the nationwide network of trained providers I've spoken of. Her staff has also expressed appreciation that her moods and memory were back to normal!

Testosterone and estrogen, as well as thyroid hormones, are vital components of the chronic pain conversation, for many reasons that may surprise you. Chronic pain and the resulting opioid crisis have been a focus for healthcare providers and lawmakers for several years. Healthcare providers who are in the chronic pain space and abreast of the published studies over the past decade regarding hormones and their relationship to chronic pain and vice versa, are seeking advanced education and training in the hormone arena and rightly so. Since 2010, multiple clinical studies speak to the relationship between pain perception and the endocrine system.

So, what causes decreased sex hormones in the pain population? Severe or low-grade chronic pain leads to insufficiency of the pituitary gland that, over time, impacts the secretion of sex hormones.

The pituitary gland is considered the master controller of all hormones and resides in the brain. The generation of pain, its transmission through the nervous system and the perception of pain by the brain, are associated with the endocrine system. There are many hormones and many factors at play in this complex "endocrine/opioid system," but a key concept to understand is that hormone decline is closely associated with chronic pain and chronic pain syndromes. Severe uncontrolled pain causes changes in the central nervous system, and constant persistent uncontrolled pain over time exerts enough stress on the "master" glands in the brain to cause inadequate secretion of testosterone and estrogen from the adrenals, ovaries, and the testicles (also known as the gonads).

"Hormone decline is closely associated with chronic pain and chronic pain syndromes."

The second most common cause of sex hormone decline in the pain population is opioid administration itself. Low testosterone levels have been observed with the administration of oral and injectable opioid pain medications. Low testosterone levels are primarily caused by the suppression of a key hormone, gonadotropin-releasing hormone, that is released by the brain and stimulates the testicles and the ovaries to secrete testosterone into the system. Opioids also can directly impair testosterone production in the adrenal glands and the gonads. Both opioid medications and the opioids that are naturally made in our body regulate the function of the gonads, primarily by acting on receptors in the brain.

Pain medications in the opioid class have multiple negative effects on the endocrine system, and this fact is vital for healthcare providers to understand when they are prescribing these medications.

In fact, one study showed androgen deficiency is evident in up to 86 percent of users, both male and female. Part of the "opioid crisis" in America is caused not only by the direct dependence resulting from chronic use of these medications, but also the vicious cycle of testosterone deficiency and hormone disruption, which exacerbates pain and decreases quality of life in all the other areas previously discussed regarding testosterone.

"Pain medications in the opioid class have multiple negative effects on the endocrine system, and this fact is vital for healthcare providers to understand when they are prescribing these medications."

Depression, anxiety, mood swings, fatigue, and an overall decreased sense of well-being add to the already depressed system of chronic pain patients and chronic pain patients on opioids. Opioids have a negative effect on thyroid-stimulating hormone from the brain, resulting in decreased levels of circulating-thyroid hormone. Low thyroid symptoms overlap with low testosterone symptoms and can include depression, fatigue, brain fog, memory loss, weight gain, and a host of negative symptoms. Other biological hormones that play active roles in pain processing are DHEA and melatonin. More on those vital hormones later.

Another aspect of chronic and acute pain that is addressed with hormones is their role as powerful anti-inflammatory molecules. Other studies have shown at the level of an injury, much like in strokes and heart attacks, there is a rapid local production of estrogen via aromatase, and estrogen down-modulates pain signaling and increases pain threshold, fancy terms for decreasing the pain a person feels after an injury.

Further, testosterone improves bone and muscle mass, directly impacting a healthy skeleton; improves energy and stamina, directly impacting the desire get to up and move about (a.k.a. exercise); decreases joint pain through its lubricating and anti-inflammatory effects and decreases recovery time after exercising.

In my practice, countless men and women share that when they started hormone therapy, their joint pain and vague aches and pains resolved; when their hormones wore off, the pain began creeping back. One patient of mine always knows when it is time to get his hormone pellets; when he plays basketball, his knees begin to ache, a telltale sign his testosterone levels are waning.

Whether you suffer from minor aches and pains, knee creaking while going up and down stairs, or chronic pain, it is essential all persons suffering from pain syndromes, whether they are on opioid medications or not, find a healthcare provider who understands how to address all of the hormone insufficiencies for optimal health, wellbeing, and quality of life.

TESTOSTERONE AND SEXUAL FUNCTION

A discussion about hormones would not be complete without addressing the issue of sexual function, or sexual dysfunction in the case of hormone decline. Susan, a 43-year-old wife and mother of three, came to my office at the prodding of her girlfriends after a discussion of hormones and sex drive came up at her neighborhood book club meeting. Many of the women in the group were raving about their improved sex lives since they had started on testosterone therapy and sharing how they were experiencing a new "honeymoon phase" with their spouses. You see, Susan had been struggling with depression, fatigue, insomnia, and low libido for about four years. She noted it started in her early 30s after her first child and worsened with her subsequent two children. When she brought the subject up to her gynecologist, she was placed on an antidepressant for her symptoms and told to return a year later for her annual exam.

Three years later, still on the antidepressants and now on sleeping pills to boot, she suffered from the common side effects of weight gain and worsening libido, and her depression had not improved. She described her outlook on life as not really depressed but more like she just didn't care (that sounds depressed to me!). This really disturbed her because she shared her children were lovely and healthy, and her husband was attentive and devoted. She said, "I have no reason to feel this way; my life is great." The weight gain further put her in a vicious cycle of lacking a desire for intimacy because she was very self-conscious about her changing body. Her depressed affect and lack of desire for any kind of intimacy with her spouse had been causing marital problems, and this was what prompted her, after listening to her girlfriends in the neighborhood, to make an appointment at my clinic.

After reviewing a thorough bloodwork analysis and medical history, it was clear she indeed had very low testosterone, non-detectable on her blood test, as well as some other hormone and nutritional deficiencies. Her treatment plan included testosterone therapy with hormone pellets and a few other things to optimize her hormone receptor activity. I also began to wean her off the antidepressants and sleeping pills, as I was certain the root cause of her moods, lack of sleep, libido, and other issues was related to her low testosterone. Five weeks later at her follow-up visit, she was a completely different person. A light sparked in her eyes that was not there at her first visit and she was astounded at the changes she was already experiencing. Her husband was also quite relieved and was amazed at the difference. He said, like many other husbands have throughout the years, "Thank you for giving me my wife back!"

This is one story of thousands of stories I could share regarding intimate relationships reigniting after getting to the root cause of the lack of sexual desire, fatigue, and depressed moods. It is a common, and very sadly under-addressed issue, for women. Sexual desire and a satisfying sex life are key components of healthy relationships, no matter the age. Multiple studies speak to the overall greater sense of wellbeing and zeal for life when sexual intimacy is a regular factor of a person's lifestyle. One researcher considers sexual health to be an additional "vital sign" when a healthcare provider is evaluating a person's overall health. I wholeheartedly agree with that sentiment!

"Sexual desire and a satisfying sex life are key components of healthy relationships, no matter the age."

Sexual dysfunction primarily is an issue for females, and erectile dysfunction is the primary sexual issue for males. Loss of sexual desire and libido in males is less common than females, but the decrease in ability to perform as the decades go by is an important aspect of male sexual aging that causes frustration and decreased intimacy. The issue of sexual dysfunction in women has been described as a huge gender gap. Much research and attention has been given to male sexual desire and erectile function, but research around female sexual dysfunction, officially termed hypoactive sexual desire disorder or HSDD, is lacking. Further compounding the issue of sexual dysfunction for females is the less-often-talked-about, but very important issue, of the inability to reach climax, termed anorgasmia.

A 2009 study reported over 16 million women over 50 have reported low sexual desire. I believe the number is much higher and spans across the age spectrum for females, most notably starting after childbearing and specifically the second child. What's fascinating about this report is although the researchers noted that the problem improved when women were placed on testosterone therapy, critics of testosterone use in women questioned the significance of this issue and therefore the report, unfortunately, has not received much attention in the medical community. It is baffling to me why so much money and effort is spent helping men achieve and maintain erections but there is little support for the female counterpart to reach a desire level to take advantage of his improved sexual function! It makes no sense to me, and frankly, addressing erectile function in a male without addressing libido in the female is a huge reason for marital discord, relationship strife, and subsequent divorces .

When testosterone levels decline, whether it is age-related, childbearing-related, or related to being on birth control pills, not only do women suffer from depression and mood alterations but also fatigue and extremely low libido. The issue for women is complex, but the solutions can be rather simple. There are vascular issues with decreased blood flow to the female sexual organs that decreased desire and ability to climax; the psychological aspect of depressed mood, lack of sleep, changing body composition, and the accompanying insecurities also impact desire and ability to climax. The neurological and physiological function of the female sex organs that change with aging cause decreases in lubrication, thinning of the vaginal wall, which causes pain, making it more difficult to stimulate a woman to climax and further decreases her desire for sex. Combine this with the male counterpart who is also aging, has decreased blood flow, and decreased ability to achieve and maintain an erection—this is a recipe for sexual disaster!

The side effects of all too commonly prescribed medications compound the issue of desire for women and desire and erectile function for men. Antidepressants are the primary culprit for women, and some blood pressure and cholesterol medications affect erectile function in men. There are also lifestyle factors, such as weight, alcohol intake, and lack of exercise that negatively impact desire and sexual function—many of those issues can also be addressed by addressing testosterone deficiency in women and men.

Every study found in women with HSSD reported resolution of symptoms with testosterone therapy. A 2015 study on the topic concluded that sexual problems were more common in women who did not use hormone therapy, notably testosterone, and another study on female sexual dysfunction concluded the problem is most likely irreversible without hormone therapy. Besides testosterone for sexual problems, there are other technologies that I have found to be highly beneficial, especially for vaginal lubrication, and the ability to climax. Treatments like laser vaginal rejuvenation, and injections to regenerate nerve tissue related to arousal are highly beneficial for these issues.

Over the last 14 years I have personally observed what optimized testosterone levels can do for men and women. I have also researched this area extensively, and many clinical studies agree, testosterone plays an active role for men and women to maintain healthy sex organs and a healthy mental outlook, improves sleep, exercise tolerance, and metabolism, and gives an overall improved vitality and sense of wellbeing.

Recap common symptoms of low testosterone for both women and men:

Depression

Anxiety

Mood swings, irritability

Insomnia

Difficulty focusing or concentrating

Brain fog, decreased mental clarity

Chronic pain

Joint pain

Muscle loss

Pain after exercise

Belly fat

Low sex drive

Sexual or erectile dysfunction

CHAPTER 6

THYROID

"Reproductive hormones aren't the only hormones that affect how you look and feel and think. Among the most influential are the hormones produced by your thyroid gland. Too little thyroid, and you feel like a slug. Hypothyroidism makes you feel like you just want to lie on the couch all day with a bag of chips. Everything works slower, including your heart, your bowels, and your brain."

Daniel G. Amen, MD

The quote above from Dr. Amen says a lot. It is so important not to have tunnel vision when it comes to optimizing these life-giving molecules called hormones. That would be like buying a classic car and only ever checking the oil and replacing the oil. You must look at all the parts of the engine and keep every single aspect of that engine running smoothly to optimize performance. The human body is no different, and unfortunately, Western medicine has evolved into a specialist-driven, symptom-treating methodology without looking at the entire body as a whole.

When you take it down to the cellular level, talking about hormones, you not only need to pay attention to the sex hormones discussed thus far, but you must also look at thyroid hormones as well as an important adrenal hormone called DHEA. The conversation wouldn't be complete without also looking at a very important hormone secreted by the brain called melatonin. Every single one of these hormones, and their precursors and downstream metabolites, play a functional, synergistic role in total physical, mental, and emotional health.

"Low thyroid doesn't kill you. It just makes you wish you were dead."
Daniel G. Amen

Every time I embark on researching and teaching about a new hormone, I think, "This one is my favorite!" Testosterone was my favorite until I needed estrogen, and then estrogen was my favorite until I discovered the benefits of thyroid, specifically raising the active thyroid hormone triiodothyronine, or T3, into an optimal, youthful range.

Thyroid hormones are metabolic hormones that are essential for life. T3 plays a crucial role in regulating mitochondrial function. Mitochondria are small, specialized organelles within cells that are often referred to as the "powerhouses" of the cell because they generate most of the cell's energy in the form of adenosine triphosphate (ATP). The close interplay between thyroid hormones and mitochondria is crucial for maintaining cellular energy homeostasis and metabolic balance throughout the body.

Thyroid hormones also regulate the basal metabolic rate, which is the amount of energy expended by the body at rest. They increase the metabolic rate by stimulating the production and activity of mitochondria. This increase in mitochondrial activity leads to enhanced ATP production and greater energy expenditure.

Thyroid hormones protect against memory loss, mood disorders like anxiety and depression, heart disease and elevated cholesterol levels, improves energy and metabolism, and impacts weight gain and weight loss, as well as the dreaded metabolic syndrome—just to name a few. Symptoms of thyroid insufficiency are fatigue and weakness, feeling cold all the time (especially the hands and feet), dry, thinning hair, thin skin and nails, and loss of the outer third of the eyebrows, loss of energy and motivation, loss of memory, depressed mood, menstrual cycle irregularities, infertility, and GI disorders like constipation. Unfortunately, so many people suffer from many of these symptoms, but when their bloodwork is done by their primary care provider, they are typically told their thyroid is "in the normal range." This is a key area

"So many people suffer from many of these symptoms, but when their bloodwork is done by their primary care provider, they are typically told their thyroid is "in the normal range."

I want to focus on re-educating you, the reader, so you are armed with great information, and you may find a healthcare provider who will treat your insufficient thyroid, regardless of what your TSH lab test shows.

UNDERSTANDING THYROID BLOOD TESTING

First, I want to talk about the thyroid lab test so you can understand what each one means for yourself.

TSH, short for thyroid-stimulating hormone, is a hormone released by the brain that goes up or down in response to circulating thyroxine (T4) levels, the primary thyroid hormone that is released from the thyroid gland. When the TSH is high, this is an indication that a patient's T4 production is low; it is an inverse or opposite relationship. If TSH is low or suppressed, this suggests adequate T4 secretion from the thyroid gland or the thyroid medication is working effectively.

A huge mistake healthcare providers make is they utilize the TSH after the patient has already started on a thyroid hormone medication. This is an erroneous use of this test. The test is simply designed to be used as a screening tool for low thyroid disease (hypothyroidism) or overactive thyroid disease (hyperthyroidism) that needs further investigation.

Once a healthcare provider starts a patient on a thyroid hormone medication, the TSH is no longer valid as a useful tool to manage their thyroid status. The only hormones that need to be checked and monitored after you begin a thyroid medication are the T4 and T3, and the most important level is the free T3.

Thyroid insufficiency vs. deficiency

There is a huge difference between thyroid deficiency and thyroid insufficiency, and it is important to understand the difference between the two when discussing thyroid hormone status. When a patient is deficient in thyroid hormone, the TSH screening test, the T4 and the free T3 will indicate the patient has what is called primary hypothyroidism. However, there are a few other cases, and they present much more frequently when the bloodwork is in the "normal reference range" but the patient is still having all the symptoms of low thyroid.

"There is a huge difference between thyroid deficiency and thyroid insufficiency, and it is important to understand the difference between the two when discussing thyroid hormone status."

Deficiency means exactly that; the thyroid hormone production is deficient, which will typically show up on a TSH lab result. Type-1 hypothyroidism, or primary hypothyroidism, is when the thyroid gland is not producing enough thyroid hormone; it is a deficient state.

Insufficiency refers to the fact that the body is making enough T4 hormone, but it is insufficient in its conversion to the active hormone, T3. There are two primary causes of thyroid insufficiency: type-2 hypothyroidism, also called non-thyroidal illness syndrome (NTIS), and type-3 hypothyroidism, which refers to receptor site resistance. Type-2 hypothyroidism is when you have a decreased conversion of T4, the primary hormone released by the thyroid gland, to the active thyroid hormone T3. *T3 is the only thyroid hormone that exerts its action on the cell.* It is vital to understand that the T3 level in the serum does not impact the TSH screening test. So, you can have a low T3 level and a normal TSH. This is the most common clinical scenario I see in practice: patients who have all the symptoms of low thyroid but their TSH is in the "normal" range, and the free T3 test—if it was even checked by the provider—is in the "low-normal" reference range. I'll speak more later why the "low-normal" reference range is not optimal for your health when referring to blood hormone levels.

Type-3 hypothyroidism, or receptor site resistance, is a rarer condition and difficult to diagnose—at the time of this writing, there is no specific lab value to test for it. It is primarily described as an insufficient stimulation of the thyroid hormone receptor. Thyroid hormone receptors are the flags on a cell that the free T3 attaches to exert its action inside the cell. Thyroid hormone receptors are present in every body system: cardiac, neurological, bones, reproductive, etc. The patient's bloodwork can present as hypo- or hyper-thyroid or normal. Recent studies suggest there is a genetic variant at the receptor level, but more research is needed to understand how to identify and manage these patients. For now, treatment depends on what symptoms they are presenting; if symptoms of low thyroid are present, treatment with a combination of thyroid medications is warranted, or if high thyroid symptoms are evident, managing with other non-thyroid medications will be necessary.

There have been a plethora of medical papers published that speak to the importance of looking at the downstream effects of thyroid hormone metabolism and paying closest attention to the active and available thyroid hormone, free T3. A person can have a normal TSH and normal T4, but their

T3 is either low or on the very end of the low range. This can happen for a variety of reasons. First and foremost, there is an age-related decrease in the conversion of T4 to T3 that typically happens after age 40, but sometimes sooner. Dietary and lifestyle factors, as well as key nutrient deficiencies also play a role in this decline in the rate of conversion.

Total T3 is all the T3 circulating in the body. Free T3 simply means the amount of T3 circulating in the body that is not bound up by other proteins or "free" to be used at the cellular level by the body. Free T3 is commonly referred to as the "active" thyroid hormone.

T3 AND THE DEIODINASE ENZYMES

There are so many things people are exposed to and do to their bodies daily that decrease production of a key enzyme called deiodinase 1. Deiodinase 1 is the primary enzyme that converts T4 to the active T3.

To name a few: physical and emotional stress, depression, extreme low-calorie dieting, insulin resistance, inflammation from an autoimmune disease or chronic disease, chronic pain, chronic fatigue and fibromyalgia, iron deficiency, exposure to toxins, and one of the most important ones that gets overlooked in the medical community so often is the synthetic drug levothyroxine. This is why so many patients on levothyroxine have "normal thyroid labs" (a.k.a. TSH) and feel terrible. If the provider were to look beyond the TSH test and look at the downstream free T3 level, that provider would see the patient's free T3 is in the lower end of the range or even below the reference range. If the provider would check another important blood test called reverse T3, that provider would also see when a patient is on levothyroxine, their reverse T3 levels are high. Why is this important? Well, reverse T3 takes that T3 and converts it back into T4! So, the body is in this continuous loop of making the active T3 hormone and then converting it to the inactive T4 hormone.

The patient feels terrible.

Other things that can increase the deiodinase 3 enzyme, the enzyme responsible for making reverse T3, are physical and emotional stress and calorie-restrictive dieting. I had a patient many years ago reach out to me to ask for help with her daughter who was having what she believed to be some strange hormonal symptoms. Her daughter was a senior in high school, a select soccer player, and had an eating disorder. She put herself through extreme calorie-restriction dieting, as well as placed very high expectations on herself from the perspective of her athletic and academic goals. In reviewing her bloodwork, it was found that her TSH and T4 were completely normal, but her free T3 was very low, which explained all her symptoms. She suffered from extreme fatigue, lethargy, depression, constipation, temperature dysregulation, menstrual cycle disruption, and a host of others. When her reverse T3 level was checked, it was incredibly high. This is because the physical and emotional stress she had put herself under was causing her body to go haywire!

Her treatment plan included coaching her on how and why this occurred, emphasizing that the expectations and stress she put on her body caused her to feel the way she did was paramount. Counseling for her eating disorder and temporarily putting her on thyroid medication until everything settled back down were also key aspects of her treatment plan. If her healthcare provider did not look at the vital downstream effects of conversion of her T4 to the active T3 hormone, it would have been completely missed. This is an unfortunate scenario I see too often in my clinical practice.

There are more reasons to pay attention to your free T3 and maintain it in the optimal range than just how you feel. But let's first talk about laboratory reference ranges. In 1998, the Clinical Laboratory Improvement Amendment, put forth by the US Food and Drug Administration, required laboratories to verify if their reference intervals or their "normal values" were appropriate for the patient population being tested. That sounds great in theory but considering the patient population being tested are Americans whose health ranges across the spectrum, it would stand to reason that the numbers on the upper end of that reference range would represent the healthiest individuals when you are speaking about laboratory markers for hormones. In other words, when you have a reference range, let's take free T3, for instance, and your range is 2.3 to 4.3, the bell curve average is going to be somewhere in the middle, around 3.0. But the upper end of that range is going to be considered healthier, optimal, or youthful levels.

Consider when you were in high school and you were taking a final exam; would you want to be on the low end or average of the bell curve of your class, or did you strive to be on the upper end of that bell curve? Everyone wants to do well in school and get good grades, but it takes work. Just like being healthy and taking care of your body takes work. Now that you understand the importance of having your free T3 tested and ensuring free T3 is in the upper limits of the range, take a look at some clinical studies that underscore the importance of these facts.

T3: THE MASTER THYROID HORMONE

As you are likely beginning to understand, T3 is the most important thyroid hormone, and free T3 levels are the most important lab test to truly assess thyroid status. Also, remember you want that free T3 level on the "right" side, literally, of the bell curve. Why? Because a free T3 in the upper end of the range is associated with better health and longevity. This is a very important concept to understand when looking at the impact that thyroid has on every single body system. Most people believe thyroid hormone is simply for metabolism, and the symptoms of thyroid deficiency are typically weight gain, thinning hair, cold hands and feet, and constipation. But what about the impact of low free T3 on other body systems that may not present with symptoms until it's too late? For example, the heart. T4 to T3 conversion happens primarily in the liver, kidneys, and skeletal muscle, but not the heart muscle.

"T3 is the most important thyroid hormone, and free T3 levels are the most important lab test to truly assess thyroid status."

The muscle cells of the heart, cardiomyocytes, are some of the few cell types that do not convert T4 to the active T3. The heart needs free T3 in the bloodstream to function properly! The impact of a low/low-normal free T3 on the heart may show up as a decreased heart rate, lower blood pressure, fatigue and pain or body-aches, known as myalgias, high cholesterol, and a general feeling of "puffiness." These are not obvious symptoms, but many people suffer from them on a daily basis. Moreover, what is the first thing most people are prescribed when a blood test shows high cholesterol?

Cholesterol-lowering medication! I wonder if anyone is thinking about looking at the free T3 level of that patient with high cholesterol? There is a root cause for every alteration in every body system, and the root cause for high cholesterol is definitely not the deficiency of a statin drug! There are many studies that show a direct correlation between a low or low-normal free T3 and increased cardiac disease or death from a cardiac disease. In one study looking at over 500 patients with heart disease, the overall death rates were five times higher in the patients with a low T3.

Another study showed a relationship between low free T3 levels and incidence of heart failure and death from heart failure. In another paper, the authors were looking at the association of low free T3 and death rates in critically ill patients on ventilators in the ICU. It was noted that patients with a free T3 below 2.3 had 52 percent higher death rate than patients with a free T3 in the middle to high reference ranges. In a research study looking at cardiovascular disease and cardiac death rates, it was noted the patients who had a free T3 level in the lower third of the reference range had higher rates of cardiac death and death from all causes (all-cause mortality) than people with a T3 in the upper third of the reference range. Again, I can't express enough, normal is NOT optimal! You see, the patients in this study all had T3 levels in the "normal" range, but they were on the wrong side of the bell curve, and the death rates of that group were significantly higher. I'm not sure about you, but I am going for my T3 in the upper third of the laboratory reference range!

What about the brain? Low free T3 is often associated with an increased risk of Alzheimer's dementia, but in this study, looking at patients in a memory clinic over the course of three years, researchers noted that neither TSH nor T4 were associated with progression of dementia to Alzheimer's disease, only the free T3. Again, if your healthcare provider is only checking the TSH—which the majority do—they will be missing critical information owing to the health of your vital organ systems!

"If your healthcare provider is only checking the TSH—which the majority do—they will be missing critical information owing to the health of your vital organ systems!"

Depression has long been associated with low thyroid, and psychiatrists have treated depression with thyroid hormones for decades. In studies over the past five years, it was noted that low T3 levels are significantly associated with higher rates of depression and insomnia, and they further stated that a blood-free T3 level could be a lab value for assessing for and predicting risk of future depression. The authors concluded that more attention needs to be paid to free T3 levels in mental healthcare.

Chronic pain is an issue of great importance in our country, and there's a direct correlation between the use of opioid pain medications and the suppression of thyroid hormone production. Chronic pain patients would do well to be assessed for low testosterone and other sex hormones as well as thyroid hormone.

What about the side effects of a "suppressed TSH"?

Remember, the TSH is released based on a feedback loop of circulating T4 levels. When T4 is high, or optimal, the TSH will be low. When T4 is low, TSH will be higher because the brain is trying to stimulate the thyroid to make more thyroid hormones. The TSH is a screening lab to assess for low or high thyroid in a patient NOT on thyroid medication. An important concept to understand when discussing thyroid hormones and thyroid lab tests is this misnomer that a low TSH on thyroid medication will have the same consequences as a low TSH from Graves' disease.

Graves' disease is an autoimmune disorder that is the primary cause of hyperthyroidism or too much thyroid hormone production. The other cause of too much thyroid hormone production is a nodule on the thyroid gland that is secreting intermittent massive amounts of thyroid hormone independent of the influence of TSH. Unfortunately, many healthcare providers have assumed the negative effects of hyperthyroid from Graves' or thyroid nodules will also apply to a low TSH level because of thyroid medication.

I have had many patients whose thyroid was functioning optimally. They felt great, their free T3 was in the upper end of the reference range, but their TSH was "low," below 1.0, only to have their primary care provider tell them their thyroid levels were way too high, and they were going to end up with a fatal arrhythmia or some other problem of hyperthyroidism. When I would ask these patients if their healthcare provider checked any of their other thyroid hormones, the answer was almost always no, and if they did check another hormone level, it was typically the T4 level. They were simply basing the misinformation on a suppressed TSH level. It's so important to understand that once you start therapy, the screening TSH test is of no use; you must look at T4 levels, T3, and free T4 and T3 levels, and sometimes free T3 to free T4 ratios.

Too many providers will erroneously believe that a suppressed TSH on therapy is going to cause atrial fibrillation, cardiac arrhythmia, osteoporosis, or other consequences of Graves' disease-related hypothyroidism. Study after study has shown that suppressed TSH on therapy does not result in any serious adverse effects, especially when the free T3 to T4 ratios are optimal. If fact, multiple studies over the past five years have shown that a high T3:T4 ratio is associated with better health outcomes. From the brain to the heart to the gut, patients with higher free T3 levels just do better overall in the areas of disease prevention and recovery from diseases and illness. In a large recently published study, it was shown that the opposite was also true: high free t4 with low free t3 level, a high T4:T3 ratio, correlated with higher all-cause mortality (death) rates and higher cardiovascular death rates. Moral to the story: make sure your healthcare provider is looking at all your thyroid hormones, including free T3 and free T4, and not just the TSH level.

TYPES OF THYROID MEDICATIONS

Levothyroxine, one of the most prescribed medications in the US, was first made in the late 1920s but became more frequently prescribed in the US in the early 1960s. It is a synthetic form of T4 or thyroxine. Synthroid is the brand name many people recognize, and its name speaks of the synthetic nature of the drug ("syn"- synthetic, "throid"- thyroid). Before T4-only preparations, also called monotherapy, came to market desiccated, often referred to as "natural" thyroid, was the mainstay of treating low thyroid conditions. Desiccated thyroid, commonly referred to as combination therapy, was the mainstay of thyroid therapy for over 60 years and includes not only T4 and T3 in the same ratios as produced by the thyroid gland, but also T2, T1, and calcitonin, also produced in the thyroid gland. These are all very important molecules for thyroid function at the cellular level.

T2 plays a vital role in the conversion of T4 to T3 via the deiodinase enzyme I spoke of earlier in this chapter. T1 one is only recently being well studied but has been found to be important for brain function and electrical activity in the brain. A hypothesis (educated guess) of one action of T1 is to counteract or keep the T4 hormone actions "in check." It's exciting to realize there is so much more to learn about these important molecules!

It all makes sense when you understand the differences between synthetic preparations of T4 and T3 compared to desiccated thyroid preparations, particularly when speaking about the patient experience. Countless studies have shown, when given a choice, most patients prefer combination therapy over monotherapy.

T he practitioners in my clinics and I combined treat more than 1000 hormone patients per month; approximately 50 percent are on desiccated thyroid hormone therapy, and many were switched from their synthetic T4. The results are always astounding. More energy, better mental focus, decreased depression, warm hands and feet, hair growth, better bowel function, and eventually weight loss occur, none of which they felt with monotherapy of synthetic T4. Among the thousands of patients I have switched to desiccated thyroid, only a handful have said they "felt better" on synthetic T4 over desiccated thyroid. It does happen, but it is very rare.

Despite those rare cases, the research has concluded patients prefer combination therapy over monotherapy to an overwhelming degree, and patients of prescribers who use combination therapy report higher treatment and practitioner satisfaction. In an interesting research study, the authors stated that although patients preferred combination therapy in the areas of mood, fatigue, wellbeing, and brain function, they could not explain why the satisfaction ratings favored the combination over monotherapy! Yes, you read that right—even though patients reported how much better they felt, and their brains worked, the researchers could not explain why the study subjects liked the combination therapy better. So, why don't more prescribing clinicians globally use more desiccated thyroid? The answer is simple. Follow the money!

It makes sense, though, if I can optimize my thyroid hormone levels as close as possible to what my body was making before age and a toxic world changed things, of course I will feel better than just replacing a part of the clinical picture .

HASHIMOTO'S THYROID

Hashimoto's thyroiditis, also known as autoimmune thyroiditis (inflammation of the thyroid), has been a topic of research for over 70 years. It is an autoimmune condition, meaning the body creates antibodies against and attacks itself, that has several theories of origin. Genetic predisposition is one known factor, but also environmental factors, dietary factors such as leaky gut (more on this later) and nutritional deficits such as selenium, are also known to cause auto-antibody production. The condition is often missed, as most healthcare providers do not routinely screen for TPO antibodies, elevations of which are hallmark to the condition.

The symptoms patients may complain of are like low thyroid: fatigue, cold intolerance, pain syndromes, depression, and other vague complaints. If the healthcare provider checks "thyroid labs," they are most often considered in the "normal range," and patients are mismanaged because they end up with prescriptions that treat the symptoms with antidepressants, pain medications, etc., rather than addressing the root cause.

The primary treatment for Hashimoto's is replacing thyroid hormone with medication, but attention to nutritional deficiencies and an evaluation of intestinal permeability (a.k.a. leaky gut), and food sensitivities is paramount; selenium deficiency is a known root cause of Hashimoto's. Often patients with Hashimoto's thyroid disease will have other autoimmune conditions, such as rheumatoid arthritis, eczema, or psoriasis—all of which the root cause could be a leaky gut. Fix the gut, fix the hypersensitive immune response and inflammation.

One last thought on sub-optimal thyroid function. In many cases, especially in younger patients who don't necessarily want to start thyroid medications, simply supplementing with selenium, iodine, zinc, and ensuring their ferritin levels are greater than 70 will often improve thyroid production. Iodine is an essential micronutrient for thyroid hormone production, and contrary to popular belief, iodine is needed and safe to be used in Hashimoto's thyroiditis; more on that in the nutrient section of this book.

CHAPTER 7

DHEA

DHEA, short for dehydroepiandrostone, is another very important hormone to our overall health. It is considered a neurosteroid because it is synthesized in the central nervous system. Historically DHEA was thought to simply be a precursor hormone for estrogen and testosterone. It is now well-known that DHEA has several of its own receptors, most notably in the brain. DHEA and its sulfate form, DHEA-S, is the most abundant circulating steroid hormone in humans. It is primarily produced in the adrenal gland, but it is also produced in the gonads (the ovaries and the testicles), as well as the brain and placenta. As with most of our hormones, there is a significant age-related decline that begins in our 30s and advances with every decade. DHEA decline has profound effects on overall human health. Interestingly, DHEA sulfate levels are approximately three times higher than total testosterone and five times higher than free testosterone! Moreover, the age-related decline of DHEA-S by up to 90 percent is more pronounced than the decline of testosterone.

DHEA, INFLAMMATION AND IMMUNITY

DHEA has several very important functions in the human body. It is considered an immunomodulator, meaning it has profound impact on our immune system and production of our natural killer T cells and other immune cells that help fight off infection. It improves physical and mental wellbeing, helps with muscle strength and bone density, and plays a role in body fat and skin elasticity because it stimulates collagen and oil production, both of which are vital to youthful, vibrant skin. DHEA at higher doses has been shown to induce remission in many patients with inflammatory bowel disease, as well as effectively treating lupus when combined with usual therapy. DHEA impacts the cardiovascular system through an anti-inflammatory response, as well as a relaxation of the arteries and vessels. Low levels have been correlated with increased heart disease and risk of all causes of death. It has also been shown to be protective of asthma and allergies because of its action on the T-helper cells and immune system.

DHEA also has been shown in several studies to decrease depression and memory loss associated with cognitive decline, as well as improve libido, especially in women. I have seen this in my clinical practice across multiple scenarios.

"DHEA also has been shown in several studies to decrease depression and memory loss associated with cognitive decline, as well as improve libido, especially in women."

One story sticks out in my mind of a lady whose husband brought her in because she suffered from extreme depression, fatigue, body aches, and brain fog—just to name a few. Her treatment included restoring her testosterone to optimal levels, addressing nutritional deficiencies and optimizing her thyroid. Because I like to use a layered approach, I held the DHEA discussion for a future office visit. I saw her again three months later, and although she reported 80 percent improvement in her symptoms, she still was battling with mild depression and some brain fog. Her DHEA was in the double digits, DHEA-S levels are optimal in women around 200 to 250 and in men, 300 to 350.

Remember that right side of the bell curve I spoke about? Those numbers are on the right side of the bell curve average. What I have found is patients who have levels in the double digits have been suffering from extreme stress typically for quite some time, which compounds the age-related decline in DHEA levels. Because this patient's DHEA levels were in the 50s, I prescribed 10 mg of a compounded DHEA supplement. I prefer a compounded supplement because, experientially, they tend to be more potent than over-the-counter DHEA supplements. At her next visit, she expressed how she couldn't believe that little daily capsule made such a profound difference in her depression and her general sense of wellbeing. It was the final missing piece of her clinical picture.

DHEA AND CORTISOL

A major problem of age-related DHEA decline is that the ratio of cortisol to DHEA becomes imbalanced. This imbalance of cortisol to DHEA has been shown to have negative effects on immune function and inflammation. DHEA and cortisol produce opposing effects in the immune system. DHEA enhances the immune system, while cortisol suppresses immunity. An elevated cortisol to DHEA ratio has been associated with higher stress and psychiatric disorders, all causes of cancer, and all causes of death, metabolic syndrome, and cognitive decline.

Let's talk about stress. Stress is a prevailing modulator of immune function, meaning it has very powerful impacts on the immune system. The stress pathway, no matter the stimulus—positive or negative — results in increased inflammatory molecules in the blood, as well as cortisol, which suppresses the immune response and increases inflammatory responses. DHEA is also released in times of stress and has the opposite effect. As DHEA levels fall due to the aging process, this ability to protect your immune response rapidly reduces. Studies on patients who have been dramatically injured show supplementation with DHEA and restoring a balance to the cortisol/DHEA ratio improves wound healing, mood, bone healing and building, as well as improved mental health and wellbeing. DHEA has also been shown to balance the effects of long-term stimulation of the fight-or-flight response induced by ongoing stressful situations. DHEA also plays a direct role in age-related muscle mass decrease, also known as sarcopenia. Sarcopenia results in decreased physical activity, impairment of a healthy metabolic system, and increased death rates.

DHEA AND THE BRAIN

Depression is a worldwide debilitating phenomenon; little has been done to move the needle forward in the areas of treating depression and depressive states. Part of the reason for this is our propensity to go right to antidepressant medications for treatment rather than looking for root cause. Hormone insufficiencies have been shown in many clinical studies to be the root cause of many depressive disorders, especially in females. Because DHEA is synthesized in the brain independent from the other endocrine glands that produce our hormones, it has a positive, wide range effect on brain function. It is associated with a molecule called glutamate released in the brain, which is linked to anxiety and depression. Studies have shown there is an inverse relationship between DHEA levels and depression and fatigue, meaning the lower DHEA levels, the greater the propensity for depression and fatigue. DHEA also plays a role in several other neurotransmitters that positively influence depression. Because DHEA has antidepressant and brain-protective effects when used to treat these conditions, it could be a very novel treatment for depression and should be considered an additional therapy in patients suffering from major depressive disorder.

"Hormone insufficiencies have been shown in many clinical studies to be the root cause of many depressive disorders, especially in females."

Research on the neuroprotective effects of DHEA show it to protect against brain cell death and stimulate brain cells to undergo repair and regeneration! It has also been used in traumatic brain injury patients and has been shown to improve brain function and motor skills.

Alzheimer's disease is another neurological disease that is rapidly growing in numbers in the US and globally. DHEA has been shown to have positive brain metabolic effects that delay brain aging because of its influence on repairing the neurons in the brain. It also is a powerful antioxidant and has been shown to potentially play a role in decreasing the brain neurodegeneration that characterizes Alzheimer's dementia.

DHEA, THE HEART, AND METABOLIC SYNDROME

Metabolic syndrome is the triad of central obesity (fat around the waist), hypertension, and insulin resistance, all of which will lead to type 2 diabetes, heart disease, and stroke when left unchecked. DHEA protects against the progression of metabolic syndrome in many ways. It can aid in weight loss, decrease abdominal visceral fat (fat around the organs) and reduces belly fat. DHEA significantly reduces insulin resistance and increases insulin sensitivity, and in one study after six months of treatment with DHEA, healthy non-obese men between 50 and 65 reduced their overall fat mass by a significant measure. Studies show low DHEA levels correlate with congestive heart failure in men, and DHEA also has been shown to protect against development and progression of cardiovascular disease, improves vascular and arterial health in women and men, and positively influences vascular inflammation, which reduces the risk factors for heart disease. In a study over the course of nine years and over 1000 men, it was found that low DHEA levels predicted ischemic heart disease independently of cholesterol levels. When administered, DHEA supplementation showed a large reduction in plaques in the aorta, hardening of the arteries, also known as atherosclerosis, and significant protection against pulmonary hypertension, as well as decreasing platelet clumping, which leads to blood clots in the coronary arteries.

SUPPLEMENTING DHEA

I'm so passionate about DHEA because of all these positive benefits! DHEA is an important part of an overall hormone optimization regimen, especially in patients whose DHEA levels are on the lowest end of the bell curve average. In the US, DHEA is considered a dietary supplement, but in other countries such as Europe, it is classified as a hormone. Because DHEA is a natural hormone created in the body, it cannot be reproduced and patented as a drug; therefore, the pharmaceutical industry is reluctant to spend resources on expensive human studies. Most of the studies around DHEA have come from private and institutional sponsors. The same holds true of testosterone for women. At any rate, DHEA is commonly available as a nutrient supplement in the States over the counter.

I have seen some over-the-counter DHEA products produce nice levels of the metabolite DHEA-sulfate; however, I prefer compounded DHEA from a compounding pharmacy. When sourced from a certified compounding pharmacy, you have the assurance that the DHEA is a pure compound with little to no additives or toxins that some over-the-counter supplements may contain.

Remember, over-the-counter supplements are not a regulated industry in the States; therefore, the manufacturing and distributing company is not accountable for ensuring the purity, potency or even accuracy of the contents of the bottle. Individual patient response is varied and unpredictable, making it difficult to make firm recommendations for dosing DHEA. There are differences in the efficacy of over-the-counter DHEA versus pharmaceutical compounded DHEA. In clinical studies, doses anywhere from 25 to 400 mg a day were found to be safe. That is a very wide range of dosing, and I don't recommend starting at high doses; every patient is an individual and needs to start low and go slow while also monitoring symptom relief and/or side effects.

Many of the side effects related to DHEA are from its conversion to DHT, the active metabolite of testosterone. This can include facial hair growth and acne because of the increased oil production from DHT. In my clinic, most female patients start with 5 to 10 mg of compounded, pharmaceutical-grade DHEA, and in men, I will start with 10 to 20 mg of compounded DHEA. For over-the-counter preparations, typically twice the compounded pharmaceutical dose is a good starting point. Caution is advised, however, in raising DHEA levels consistently above the reference range. If you are going to take a DHEA supplement, it is best to take it under the care and guidance of your healthcare provider who can monitor blood levels on an annual or semi-annual basis.

CHAPTER 8

MELATONIN

"There is renewal in rest."
Lailah Gifty Akita
"Sleep is the best meditation."
Dalai Lama

Think for a moment about your lifestyle as it pertains to light stimulation. Do you fall asleep with a computer, cell phone screen, or television on in your room? Do you use a computer, cell phone, or watch television within an hour of going to bed and going to sleep? Do you have nightlights or ambient light piercing the darkness of your bedroom? Do you live in a city that never sleeps like Las Vegas? Are you a night shift worker who never gets full dark exposure?

If you answered yes to any of those questions, it's very possible your melatonin levels are suffering the consequence of continuous light stimulation. I think of all the children who go to bed with their phones, scrolling through social media or watching videos. Or the ones like my daughter who sleep with a cell phone right by their head, so every time a message or notification comes through, the light pings and disrupts her sleep.

Melatonin is a hormone produced by the pineal gland in the brain, which regulates the sleep-wake cycle. Melatonin levels naturally rise at night, signaling to the body it's time to sleep, and decrease in the morning, signaling it's time to wake up. Melatonin is essential for the regulation of sleep, but it also has other important functions in the body.

One of the most significant roles of melatonin is its ability to help regulate the immune system. Melatonin is a powerful antioxidant that can neutralize harmful free radicals, reducing oxidative stress and inflammation in the body. This antioxidant activity is particularly important for the immune system, as oxidative stress and inflammation can weaken the immune response, making it more difficult for the body to fight off infections.

In addition to its antioxidant properties, melatonin also plays a role in regulating the body's circadian rhythms. These rhythms help to regulate a wide range of bodily functions, including metabolism, hormone production, and immune system function. Disruptions to circadian rhythms can have significant negative effects on health, including increasing the risk of chronic diseases such as diabetes, cardiovascular disease, and cancer.

In my research on melatonin, I came across a very large study that showed a direct correlation between nightshift workers and increased cancer rates; this correlation has been directly linked to the decrease in melatonin production that is a consequence of nightshift working. After understanding the importance of getting supplemental melatonin for nightshift workers, I've made this a vital part of my clinical practice. Nightshift workers should be taking additional melatonin in the morning before they go to sleep but also doing everything they can to shut out all artificial light from their sleeping quarters. Blackout shades* and white noise sound machines have also been shown to be beneficial.

Melatonin also has mighty anti-inflammatory properties and can play a significant role in regulating inflammation in the body. Inflammation is a natural response of the immune system to injury, infection, or other types of damage and plays a critical role in the body's defense against pathogens. As previously discussed, chronic inflammation can lead to a range of health problems, including autoimmune disorders, cardiovascular disease, and cancer. Melatonin can help to reduce chronic inflammation by neutralizing harmful free radicals in the body and inhibiting the production of pro-inflammatory cytokines, proteins that are secreted by the immune system and other tissues.

"Chronic inflammation can lead to a range of health problems, including autoimmune disorders, cardiovascular disease, and cancer."

Melatonin also can regulate the activity of immune cells, such as T cells and B cells, which play a critical role in the immune response. Melatonin has been shown to enhance the activity of these cells and promote a more robust immune response, particularly in the context of infection. In addition to its anti-inflammatory properties, melatonin can also help to reduce oxidative stress in the body. Oxidative stress occurs when there is an imbalance between the production of free radicals and the body's ability to neutralize them, leading to cellular damage and inflammation.

Melatonin also plays a role in regulating the body's response to stress. When the body is under stress, it produces cortisol, a hormone that can disrupt the sleep-wake cycle and increase feelings of anxiety and depression. Melatonin can help to counteract the effects of cortisol, reducing feelings of stress and anxiety and promoting restful sleep. This could be one of the reasons melatonin has been shown in several studies to lower blood pressure. During 2020 and 2021, due to the plethora of studies that were coming out around melatonin and its ability to mitigate exacerbation of COVID-19 symptoms, several of my patients were taking higher doses of melatonin. Some patients were taking doses in the range of 20 to 40 mg a night, not only because they believed it would prevent them from getting severely ill, but also because they realized it took doses in that range to help their body shut down and get adequate sleep!

On several occasions, I noticed patients who struggled with chronic, mildly elevated blood pressure had normalized on the melatonin! I thought this was a very interesting coincidence until I started researching melatonin for myself. What I found was, in addition to melatonin's role on inflammation and oxidative stress, melatonin has been shown to help to regulate the activity of the sympathetic nervous system, which plays a key role in blood pressure regulation. This isn't always the case, however; some studies showed an increase in blood pressure when certain patients took melatonin. It does seem to be related to the patient's age and overall health status, as well as other medications they may be taking.

Unfortunately, in today's modern world, many people have inadequate levels of melatonin, which can lead to a range of health problems. Factors such as aging, exposure to artificial light at night, and certain medications can all disrupt the body's natural production of melatonin, leading to low levels of the hormone. This can result in sleep disturbances, weakened immune function, and increased risk of chronic disease. Like our other hormones, melatonin production naturally declines with age, with levels typically starting to decrease around age 40 and continuing to decline throughout the lifespan. Even though it may not fully wake you, the fact there is light stimulation will impact your sleep and melatonin levels. You may think you had a good night sleep, but if you wake up not feeling rested, struggle with the ability to focus, feel depressed or anxious, or have challenges fighting common colds and other infections, these may be signs you are not getting enough melatonin secretion at night.

"Factors such as aging, exposure to artificial light at night, and certain medications can all disrupt the body's natural production of melatonin."

Recap: reasons melatonin levels decline:

1. **Aging:** As people age, the body's natural production of melatonin tends to decrease, making it more difficult to fall asleep and stay asleep.

2. **Exposure to artificial light at night**: Exposure to artificial light at night can disrupt the body's natural production of melatonin by suppressing its release. This includes light from electronic devices, streetlights, and indoor lighting.

3. **Shift work or jetlag:** Disruptions to the sleep-wake cycle, such as those caused by shift work or jetlag, can alter the body's natural production of melatonin, leading to lower levels of the hormone.

4. **Certain medications:** Some medications, such as beta-blockers and benzodiazepines, can decrease the body's natural production of melatonin.

5. **Medical conditions:** Certain medical conditions, such as sleep disorders, depression, and anxiety, can disrupt the body's natural production of melatonin, leading to lower levels of the hormone.

Recap: melatonin insufficiency symptoms:

1. **Difficulty falling asleep or staying asleep:** Melatonin is essential for regulating the sleep-wake cycle, and low levels of the hormone can make it difficult to fall asleep or stay asleep throughout the night.

2. **Increased sensitivity to light:** Melatonin is produced in response to darkness and is suppressed by light. Low levels of the hormone can make individuals more sensitive to light, making it more difficult to fall asleep or stay asleep in a bright environment.

3. **Mood disturbances:** Melatonin insufficiency has been linked to an increased risk of mood disorders such as depression and anxiety. This may be due to the role of

melatonin in regulating the body's stress response and promoting restful sleep.

4. **Weakened immune function:** Melatonin plays a critical role in regulating immune function, and low levels of the hormone can lead to weakened immunity and an increased risk of infections.

5. **Increased risk of chronic diseases:** Melatonin insufficiency has been linked to an increased risk of chronic diseases such as cardiovascular disease, diabetes, and cancer due to the role of melatonin in regulating inflammation and oxidative stress in the body.

To maintain adequate levels of melatonin, it's important to prioritize healthy sleep habits. This includes getting enough sleep each night, creating a sleep-friendly environment by reducing exposure to light and noise, and avoiding stimulating activities such as using electronic devices or watching TV before bedtime. In many cases, melatonin supplements may be recommended to help boost levels of the hormone, improve sleep quality, and prevent the consequences of melatonin deficiency, such as inflammation, immunity, and stress.

Melatonin doses come in a wide range of choices. Some people are sensitive to melatonin initially and complain of extreme grogginess, even at very low doses, but this side effect decreases over time the more they are exposed to adequate amounts of melatonin. The dose choice of melatonin really depends on the person's lifestyle. If you are a night shift worker, I would suggest no less than 10 mg before sleep; if you suffer from many chronic diseases (which are all rooted in inflammation), you may need higher doses.

When suffering from viral illness, 5-20 mg may be helpful to overcome being sick. People trying to transition off sleeping medications may need higher doses in the 10-20 + ranges. The average adult, however, does well with 3-5 mg before sleep.

CHAPTER 9

GUT HEALTH & HORMONES

"Gut health is everything, it's the second brain, where many of our hormones are produced."
Tess Daly

When I am lecturing on how to optimize hormones for doctors and other healthcare practitioners, many attendees at our trainings are surprised when I open the afternoon with a lecture on gut health, diet, and nutrient supplements. Most of them thought they were just coming to learn how to diagnose hormone insufficiency and how to dose hormones appropriately in their patients. However, by the end of the lecture, it becomes abundantly clear there is a lot more to optimizing hormones than just getting blood levels on the right side of the reference range!

The best analogy I can give is having a beautiful classic car. Now, just imagine this is the car of your dreams—it doesn't even have to be a classic restored car—it can be a brand-new luxury sports car! Would you spend so much time, energy, and effort saving, researching, and looking forward to the day you can own your dream car just to get it and only ever fill the gas tank up with fuel? Would you not maintain the engine, make sure it had tune-ups and all the pistons were firing, and the engine was running smoothly? Put another way, you wouldn't just fuel your car, but you would want that fuel to burn efficiently and the car to perform at its highest level. Well, the same holds true for the human body!

In the case of hormone therapies, healthcare providers would be remiss to give a patient a hormone medication and fail to pay attention to ensuring the hormone "fuel" gets into the engine, or in this case, the cell. The hormone must get to the cell to do its work and support the incredible machine that is the human body run as efficiently as possible. Further, paying attention to how the hormones are metabolized is paramount.

There are so many nuances to optimizing hormones because the body is a unique mysterious machine that really is, what my friend Dr. James LaValle calls, "a system of systems." You have learned how hormone levels impact depression, anxiety, and other mood disorders, as well as cardiovascular disease, neurovascular diseases like strokes and Alzheimer's, cancer, diabetes, and insulin resistance. Knowing the role hormones play in so many distinct body functions and prevention of many chronic diseases, it would be negligent to leave out the impact of the gut on many of these same chronic disease processes influenced by hormone health.

This is one of the problems with Western medicine; in my opinion, the medical community has tunnel vision. Specialists focus on one area, often without giving any credence to other parts of the body that might be influencing or be influenced by those other areas. For instance, consider the continual and direct communication between the gut and the brain. For a neurologist to exclusively treat the brain as an independent organ with no influence on or from other parts of the body does not make sense. The same concept holds true for a gastroenterologist, cardiologist, endocrinologist, gynecologist, dermatologist, really any specialty area of medicine, including family and internal medicine practitioners! Every medical practitioner needs to have a firm grasp of how all our body systems work together. This symbiosis is a key aspect of health and wellness, not to mention longevity.

"One of the problems with Western medicine; in my opinion, the medical community has tunnel vision."

THE GUT

"All diseases begin in the gut."
Hippocrates

"The gut," refers to the bowels, or the intestines, also referred to as the GI (gastrointestinal) tract. This is a distinction from the stomach, where food digestion takes place. Once food is digested and moves through the intestinal tract, some incredible things start happening! But also, some pretty bad things can happen, depending on lifestyle factors such as diet, stress, exercise, toxicity—emotional and physical—which can all lead to an unhealthy gut. You may have heard the term the gut microbiome. This is a term I have been using in clinical practice for about a decade, but it is only just recently becoming accepted in mainstream medicine, and although many healthcare providers know the word, they don't really understand the importance of altering your gut microbiome to a healthy environment and the impact it has on overall health and disease prevention. Part of the reason is, it's just not taught in medical schools or any clinical training of nurse practitioners, physician's assistants, or other clinicians. For healthcare providers to learn about the intricacies of the gut and how it impacts overall health, and how to teach their patients to have a healthy gut, they must attend advanced clinical trainings that focus on a functional or integrated approach to medicine.

It is why I'm so passionate about sharing this information with you, the reader! Some of our best education as clinicians starts with our patients. That is, if practitioners take the time to listen. I have certainly learned a lot from my patients over the years who were looking for answers to their health problems that they couldn't get from their primary care providers. There is so much information available when you really sit down and ask deep, probing questions about a person's history, all the way back to childhood and even sometimes in the womb. Understanding childhood trauma, physical or emotional, and the impact it has on gut health is imperative. Sports injuries like traumatic brain injuries or concussions, even mild, can cause intestinal permeability issues, a.k.a. leaky gut—within as little as 20 minutes!

To truly illustrate this, a particular patient case comes to mind. She was a 19-year-old girl who was having extreme gastrointestinal symptoms, like bloating, stomach pain, and multiple others. She changed her diet and ate what she considered a "healthy diet" of salads and grilled fish while increasing consumption of fruits and vegetables, but she still did not feel better.

During her initial consultation, she shared details about her extremely stressful life that started in the womb. She was born into poverty of a drug-addicted mother, and the first decade of her life was spent under exceptionally poor conditions. At four years old, she describes pushing a chair up to the stove and making her own dinner, as her mother was unavailable or unable to care for her. She told stories of being a two-year-old walking down the street in a dirty diaper until someone picked her up and took her back to her home; she was profoundly neglected. She was eventually adopted in her early teenage years, but the damage was already done. Extreme stress experienced in her early developmental years had a profoundly negative impact on her mental and emotional health as well as physical health. Symptoms for this patient were rooted in her early years, starting in the womb of a stressed, malnourished, and drug-addicted mother, manifested as a "leaky gut" and caused multiple vague symptoms not only directly related to food and eating, but also depressed mood, anxiety, and difficulty focusing. After testing her for food sensitivities, my team and I found she had multiple issues that were causing her symptoms, and even the presumed "healthy" foods were causing problems because of her leaky gut.

WHAT IS A LEAKY GUT?

Leaky gut syndrome, also known as intestinal permeability, is a condition in which the lining of the small intestine becomes damaged and allows undigested food particles, toxins, and other harmful substances to "leak" into the bloodstream. This can trigger an immune response and cause inflammation throughout the body. The causes of leaky gut are related to a variety of factors, including a poor diet, chronic stress, head injuries, certain medications like antibiotics and NSAIDS like ibuprofen; as well as infections and imbalances in gut bacteria, also called gut dysbiosis. The relationship between sucralose and leaky gut is a topic that has gained some attention in recent years, but it remains a subject of debate and ongoing research. Sucralose is a non-caloric artificial sweetener commonly used as a sugar substitute in various food and beverage products. Some individuals have raised concerns that sucralose, along with other artificial sweeteners, may contribute to or exacerbate leaky gut syndrome. Some studies have suggested that artificial sweeteners, including sucralose, could also have effects on the gut microbiome.

Symptoms of a leaky gut can include: bloating, gas, abdominal pain, diarrhea, constipation, fatigue, joint pain, depression, anxiety, brain fog, ADD (attention deficit disorder), skin rashes, as well as manifestations of autoimmune disorders like Hashimoto's thyroid, eczema, psoriasis, rheumatoid arthritis, and others.

While some functional, alternative, or integrative health practitioners diagnose and treat leaky gut syndrome, the concept is not widely recognized by the medical community, even gastroenterologists, as a distinct medical condition. Because of the vague symptoms listed above, and the mainstay of Western clinical training, a leaky gut is often "treated" by symptom management with antidepressants, anti-anxiety medications, ADD medications, topical steroids, etc. You get the picture—the root cause is rarely addressed! Again, not the fault of your trained healthcare provider, it is simply that the "training" for practitioners rarely includes concepts like gut health, diet, and nutrition. More on how to heal the gut at the end of this chapter.

"Symptoms of a leaky gut can include bloating, gas, abdominal pain, diarrhea, constipation, fatigue, joint pain, depression, anxiety, brain fog, ADD (attention deficit disorder), skin rashes, as well as manifestations of autoimmune disorders like Hashimoto's thyroid, eczema, psoriasis, rheumatoid arthritis, and others."

WHAT IS GUT DYSBIOSIS?

Gut dysbiosis means an imbalance or disruption of the "good bacteria" that normally inhabits the human gut. It is also referred to as the gut microbiota or microbiome. The gut microbiota plays a crucial role in maintaining digestive and overall health by aiding in digestion, producing essential vitamins and nutrients, and supporting the immune system. The opposite of dysbiosis is eubiosis, a state of microbial balance in the body that is associated with health and prevention of many diseases.

In gut dysbiosis, the composition and diversity of the gut microbiota may be altered with an overgrowth of certain harmful bacteria and a decrease in beneficial bacteria. This imbalance can lead to various health problems, including digestive issues, inflammation, and a weakened immune system. Inflammation is the key trigger for all chronic disease processes, including heart disease, brain conditions like Alzheimer's and strokes, autoimmune disorders, asthma, and other pulmonary conditions, to name a few. There is a wealth of recent clinical data that points to an altered gut microbiome as a root cause of inflammation.

One of the known factors of inflammation originating in the unhealthy gut is lipopolysaccharides (LPS). LPS are large molecules found in the outer membranes of certain types of bacteria, including some that are commonly found in the gut microbiota. LPS are also known as endotoxins because they can cause inflammation and other harmful effects when they enter the bloodstream. Endotoxins are toxins that are present inside a bacterial cell that is released when the cell breaks down.

An imbalance in the gut microbiota can lead to an overgrowth of LPS-producing bacteria, which can increase the levels of LPS in the gut and promote gut inflammation. This can also lead to "leaky gut," as explained previously, in which the intestinal barrier becomes permeable and allows harmful substances, including LPS, to pass through into the bloodstream. Once in the bloodstream, LPS can trigger an immune response and promote inflammation throughout the body. Chronic inflammation can contribute to a range of health problems, including insulin resistance, obesity, and other metabolic disorders, as well as autoimmune diseases, neurodegenerative diseases like Alzheimer's dementia, and cardiovascular disease.

Remember the brilliance of Hippocrates centuries ago when he stated, "All diseases begin in the gut"? Turns out, he was a genius and totally correct. Modern medicine serves the medical community well in so many areas, especially stabilizing emergencies like strokes and heart attacks, but I believe the medical community has gotten so far from the basics with fancy diagnostic tools and lab tests, clinicians have neglected to pay attention to the soil in which most to all disease stems from: *an inflamed, leaky, and unhealthy gut.*

"Medical community has gotten so far from the basics with fancy diagnostic tools and lab tests, clinicians have neglected to pay attention to the soil in which most to all disease stems from: an inflamed, leaky, and unhealthy gut."

THE GUT-BRAIN CONNECTION

The relationship between gut and brain health was first postulated in the early 1900s, but only over the past decade—more than 100 years later—has research begun to focus on the gut-brain connection, also known as the gut-brain axis. The gut-brain axis refers to the communication network between the gut and the brain, which involves bidirectional (functioning in both directions) communication between the central nervous system (CNS) and the enteric (from the intestines) nervous system (ENS). The enteric nervous system is a complex network of neurons (nerve cells) and supporting cells located within the walls of the gastrointestinal tract. It is sometimes called the "second brain" because it can function independently of the central nervous system and control many digestive processes. The ENS is made up of two main layers of neurons that coordinate many aspects of gut function, including motility, secretion, and blood flow. The gut-brain axis allows for a constant flow of signals between the gut and the brain, which can influence various physiological processes, including digestion, appetite, mood, immune function, and more. For example, certain gut bacteria can produce neurotransmitters and other signaling molecules that can affect brain function and behavior, while stress and other psychological factors can affect gut motility and function.

STRESS

Here it is again! Stress! To be specific, chronic stress. Chronic mental or emotional stress often has a significant impact on the function of the ENS, which in turn can affect digestive function and overall health. During periods of chronic stress, the body releases high levels of stress hormones, including cortisol and adrenaline. These hormones can have a direct effect on the ENS by disrupting the balance of neurotransmitters in the gut, leading to digestive problems such as diarrhea, constipation, or bloating. Stress can also cause changes to gut motility, impacting the speed and movement of food through the digestive system. Stress can even trigger inflammation in the gut, further exacerbating existing gut problems or causing the development of new ones! Lastly, chronic stress can also lead to dysbiosis, which is now understood to further contribute to gastrointestinal symptoms, GI disorders like Crohn's disease and ulcerative colitis, inflammation, and effect overall health.

DEPRESSION

Depression is a worldwide phenomenon that is rapidly growing. I've discussed hormonal influences on depression, but there is growing evidence to suggest that disruptions in the gut microbiota can also contribute to the development and exacerbation of depressive symptoms through several mechanisms. One mechanism is through the production of neurotransmitters, such as serotonin and dopamine. These neurotransmitters play important roles in regulating mood and emotional wellbeing, and most of them are produced in the gut! Dysbiosis can alter the production and balance of these neurotransmitters, leading to imbalances that may contribute to depression, anxiety, and sleep disturbances that often compound the problem. The increased levels of inflammation and oxidative stress caused by dysbiosis can also contribute to the development of depression. Furthermore, dysbiosis can also affect the production of short-chain fatty acids (SCFAs), which are important for regulating immune function and reducing inflammation in the gut and the brain. Dysbiosis can reduce the production of SCFAs, which exacerbates the increased inflammation and oxidative stress.

Gut dysbiosis is now known to promote many negative consequences in the brain that lead to a host of diseases. Imbalances or disruptions in the gut-brain axis have been linked to many health problems, including irritable bowel syndrome, depression, anxiety, and other mental health disorders, as well as Alzheimer's disease and strokes. Understanding and optimizing the gut-brain axis is an important area of research for improving overall health and prevention and treatment of various brain-related health conditions.

GUT HEALTH AND IMMUNE FUNCTION

The gut microbiota plays a critical role in shaping and regulating the immune system by promoting the development of immune cells and maintaining immune homeostasis or equilibrium. Dysbiosis can lead to alterations in the gut microbiota composition and diversity, which can in turn affect immune function. One way which gut dysbiosis can impact immune function is by promoting inflammation. Dysbiosis often leads to an overgrowth of harmful bacteria, triggering an immune response and promoting inflammation throughout the body, largely via LPS as discussed earlier. This chronic inflammation is linked to a range of health problems related to an altered immune response, including autoimmune disorders, allergies, cancers, and more.

"Imbalances or disruptions in the gut-brain axis have been linked to many health problems, including irritable bowel syndrome, depression, anxiety, and other mental health disorders, as well as Alzheimer's disease and strokes."

Gut dysbiosis can also affect immune function by altering the production of certain immune cells, such as T cells and B cells, and by influencing the production of cytokines and other signaling molecules involved in immune function. Cytokines are a group of small proteins that are secreted by cells in the immune system and other tissues. They act as signaling molecules, helping to coordinate the body's immune response to infection, inflammation, and other types of stress or injury. They can have a wide range of effects on the immune system, including stimulating the production of more immune cells, increasing inflammation, or promoting the resolution of inflammation, and research has shown that restoring a healthy balance of gut microbiota can help to improve immune function and reduce inflammation.

Leaky gut syndrome and autoimmune disorders are closely related because the increased intestinal permeability associated with leaky gut can contribute to the development of autoimmune disorders. As a reminder, in leaky gut syndrome the lining of the small intestine becomes damaged, allowing undigested food particles, toxins, and other harmful substances to leak into the bloodstream. This can trigger an immune response and lead to chronic inflammation throughout the body. This chronic inflammation can eventually damage tissues and organs, leading to the development of autoimmune disorders. Autoimmune disorders occur when the immune system mistakenly attacks healthy cells and tissues in the body, leading to chronic inflammation and tissue damage. Some autoimmune disorders known to have a root cause in gut dysbiosis and leaky gut are inflammatory bowel disease, lupus, rheumatoid arthritis, multiple sclerosis, Graves' disease, Hashimoto's thyroid, and even type 1 diabetes.

Treating leaky gut syndrome and restoring a healthy balance of gut microbiota has been shown in research to reduce inflammation and improve the function of the immune system, potentially reducing the risk of developing autoimmune disorders and other immune-related issues. More on treating gut issues later.

GUT HEALTH AND THE HEART

There is growing evidence to suggest that gut dysbiosis may play a role in the development of cardiovascular disease (CVD). This can happen in several ways. One way is through the production of trimethylamine-N-oxide (TMAO), a metabolite that is produced by certain bacteria in the gut. TMAO has been shown to contribute to the development of atherosclerosis, (hardening of the arteries) a major risk factor for CVD. TMAO can also promote platelet activation and aggregation, which can lead to blood clot formation and increase the risk of heart attack and stroke. Platelets are the sticky cells that clump together to create a blood clot. They are great to have around when you cut yourself, but another story when it comes to clogging an artery!

Another way is through the promotion of chronic inflammation. Remember LPS? An imbalance in the gut microbiota can lead to the production of these pro-inflammatory molecules that contribute to systemic inflammation, a major contributor to the development of CVD. Furthermore, gut dysbiosis has been shown to contribute to metabolic dysfunction, including insulin resistance, obesity, and altered blood lipids, all of which are major risk factors for CVD.

There is also evidence to suggest that gut dysbiosis may contribute to the development and progression of congestive heart failure (CHF) through several mechanisms. The endothelium is a thin layer of cells that line the blood vessels, heart, and lymph tissues. TMAO promotes inflammation, oxidative stress, and endothelial dysfunction, and an increase in the production of these harmful metabolites can also contribute to the development of CHF. Gut dysbiosis can also contribute to the development of CHF by allowing bacteria or bacterial products to move into the bloodstream. This can trigger an immune response and inflammation, which can damage the heart and contribute to the progression of CHF.

Lastly, the LPS produced by an unhealthy gut microbiome promotes inflammation and oxidative stress in the heart and other organs, which contributes to the development of heart failure and other cardiovascular problems.

GUT HEALTH AND CANCER

The relationship between gut dysbiosis and cancer is complex. Several mechanisms have been proposed to explain how gut dysbiosis can contribute to cancer development. For example, certain bacteria in the gut produce metabolites that can damage DNA and promote the growth of cancer cells. Other bacteria may produce inflammatory molecules that can promote chronic inflammation, a known risk factor for cancer. There it is again, inflammation! Are you starting to see the picture? Chronic stress and a poor diet lead to an unhealthy gut environment, leading to chronic inflammation, which leads to all disease.

Cancer cells arise due to genetic mutations that allow them to grow and divide uncontrollably. These mutated cells can often go undetected by the immune system and continue to grow and spread throughout the body, ultimately leading to cancer. The immune system is equipped with various cells and molecules that can recognize and eliminate cancer cells. For example, white blood cells called T cells can recognize and kill cancer cells directly, while other cells called natural-killer cells can target cancer cells without the need for prior recognition.

An imbalance in the gut microbiota can lead to a weakened immune response, making it easier for cancer cells to evade detection by the immune system and multiply. Recent studies have also suggested that gut dysbiosis may be linked to an increased risk of certain types of cancer, including colorectal, liver, pancreatic, and breast cancer.

GUT HEALTH AND HORMONES

The gut microbiome is now considered to be a full-fledged endocrine, hormone-secreting organ! The gut and hormone balance are closely linked, as the gut microbiota plays an important role in regulating the production, metabolism, and balance of hormones throughout the body, such as insulin, cortisol, and the sex hormones (estrogen, progesterone, and testosterone). Additionally, gut bacteria can produce certain hormones and hormone-like substances that can influence various processes in the body.

"The gut and hormone balance are closely linked, as the gut microbiota plays an important role in regulating the production, metabolism, and balance of hormones throughout the body."

The gut and hormone balance are also connected through the gut-brain axis. This communication pathway involves the release of hormones and other signaling molecules from the gut that can influence brain function and behavior, as well as the release of hormones from the brain that can affect gut motility and function. Gut dysbiosis can lead to disruptions in hormone balance and contribute to a range of health problems, including metabolic disorders, menstrual irregularities, and fertility issues. For example, an overgrowth of harmful bacteria in the gut can lead to insulin resistance and elevated cortisol levels, which can contribute to the development of type-II diabetes and other metabolic disorders like polycystic ovarian syndrome, or PCOS, which is directly related to infertility.

Estrogen plays an important role in regulating various aspects of gut function, including gut motility, immune function, and the composition of the gut microbiota. Estrogen can influence gut motility by affecting the contraction and relaxation of smooth muscle cells in the gut wall, which can impact digestion and bowel movements. Additionally, estrogen can regulate or help balance the immune response in the gut, helping to protect against harmful pathogens while maintaining a healthy balance of gut bacteria. Furthermore, estrogen can affect the composition of the gut microbiota by promoting the growth and activity of certain bacteria that produce beneficial metabolites, such as short-chain fatty acids, that support gut health. Imbalances in estrogen levels, such as those seen during menopause, can lead to changes in gut motility, immune function, and the gut microbiota, which may contribute to digestive problems and other health issues. Estrogen deficiency, as seen after menopause in women not getting hormone replacement, has been directly linked to increased colon cancer risk.

The estrobolome refers to the collection of bacterial genes in the gut microbiome that are involved in the metabolism of estrogen. The estrobolome is thought to play an important role in maintaining hormonal balance in the body, as imbalances in estrogen metabolism have been associated with a variety of estrogen-related health issues, including breast cancer, endometriosis, and infertility. Estrogen metabolism also occurs in several phases in the liver. The process of estrogen metabolism in the liver and in the gut via the estrobolome, can be divided into two main pathways: the "good" pathway and the "bad" pathway.

The "good" pathway involves the production of estrogen metabolites that have anti-cancer properties and are less likely to cause harm throughout the body. The "bad" pathway, on the other hand, produces estrogen metabolites that can be harmful and may contribute to the development of estrogen-related health issues noted previously. In the glucuronidation phase of estrogen metabolism in the liver, the "bad" estrogen, metabolites are bound to the enzyme glucuronidase to be taken to the bowel for excretion. An overgrowth of bad bacteria in the gut (dysbiosis) causes increases of an enzyme called beta-glucuronidase. Beta-glucuronidase uncouples glucuronidase from the "bad" bacteria in the gut, and then it is reabsorbed into the bloodstream. It is now thought that the recirculation of these more carcinogenic, or cancer-causing, metabolites cause an increased risk for breast and other estrogen-related cancers.

Another key factor to consider in cancers and gut-related disorders are the so-called endocrine disruptors (EDs). Endocrine disruptors are chemicals or substances that can interfere with the normal functioning of the endocrine hormone system. Endocrine disruptors can mimic, block, or interfere with the action of hormones in the body, leading to a variety of adverse effects, such as developmental abnormalities, reproductive problems, and immune system disorders. They can also disrupt the communication between the hormones and their target cells, leading to a range of health problems, including obesity, diabetes, and cancer.

Examples of endocrine disruptors include certain pesticides, plastics, flame retardants, and even some prescription medications like birth control pills, bisphosphonates given for osteoporosis, antidepressants, and others. The chemical EDs can enter the body through food, water, air, and skin contact and can accumulate in fatty tissues, making them difficult to eliminate. A primary way many of these endocrine disruptors into our body through plastics is plastic water bottles, food containers, and packaging. Especially when exposed to heat, the harmful chemicals and plastics leach into the food or liquid that it is stored in and, when consumed, accumulates in the body.

"Endocrine disruptors are chemicals or substances that can interfere with the normal functioning of the endocrine hormone system."

Recap: What causes leaky gut and gut dysbiosis?

Remember, there is a difference between a leaky gut and an imbalanced gut microbiome (dysbiosis), yet they are essentially and importantly related. Several factors have been known to cause both a leaky gut and gut dysbiosis, many I have already mentioned but will recap a few key players:

1. **Dietary choices**
2. **Chronic stress**
3. **Age:** As people age, the diversity and abundance of beneficial gut bacteria tend to decrease
4. **Medications:** Antibiotics top the list! As well as proton pump inhibitors, given for indigestion and heartburn,

nonsteroidal anti-inflammatory drugs (NSAIDs), and the endocrine disruptors mentioned previously

5. **Exposure to toxins:** Exposure to environmental toxins, such as plastics, pesticides, and heavy metals
6. **Exposure to chemical endocrine disruptors (EDs)**

THE IMPORTANCE OF A HEALTHY DIET

I cannot express diet enough. Remember yet another quote from Hippocrates, "Let your food be your medicine." Aside from the toxic things put in our minds and on our bodies, everything put in your mouths plays a role in your gut, and subsequently your hormone health. There is a great deal of evidence that shows the Standard American Diet (notice the acronym is SAD) has an extremely negative impact on gut health. That is because the "SAD" primarily consists of calorie-dense but nutrient-deficient foods. A Western (SAD) diet is typically characterized by high intakes of processed foods, refined carbohydrates, saturated and trans fats, and low intakes of fruits, vegetables, and whole grains. This type of diet has been linked to an increased risk of several chronic diseases, such as obesity, type 2 diabetes, cardiovascular disease, and cancer.

"Aside from the toxic things put in our minds and on our bodies, everything put in your mouths plays a role in your gut, and subsequently your hormone health."

Packaged and processed foods, the use of high-fructose corn syrup, seed oils, sucralose, and other chemicals found in processed food, and mass-produced genetically modified

(GMO) foods, are the primary issues. Several different studies have shown that when people migrate from other countries to the US and adopt the Western diet and lifestyle, negative health changes in their bodies can be evident as soon as a few weeks to a few months! Coupled with the lack of fiber from the decreased number of fresh fruits and vegetables, the "SAD" Western diet is another recipe for disaster. Pun intended !

THE IMPORTANCE OF A HEALTHY MIND

A lovely young patient of mine in her 30s, married with two kids, has been seeing me for hormone optimization for a couple of years. Every time I would see her, she would report a new ailment or issue that she was seeking a specialist care for. After about a year of seeing her go from specialist to specialist in an effort to figure out what was going on, I started asking her some key questions about her life, her childhood, and her current state of mind.

I suggested that she go through our program, called the Metabolic Code®. The Metabolic Code® is an amazing functional and integrated health program, created by Dr. James LaValle, that helps practitioners dial in on less obvious, more subtle cues that a patient is suffering in some way that is impacting their physical health. After we did some special lab work, and she filled out the metabolic code questionnaire, the results gave me some key things to focus on. She had issues with her adrenals and cortisol (stress), and her gut. I asked some questions about her past regarding physical or emotional abuse, or any trauma to her head, and she shared that she had suffered many bouts of trauma and a few concussions as well as admitted, tearfully, there were some very toxic people in her life.

I started to explain to her how that type of stress- mental, physical, spiritual, and emotional- would impact her immune function, her gut, and cause a great deal of whole-body inflammation. You see the next doctor she was scheduled to see was a rheumatologist to rule out auto immune dysfunction. She did not want to go on all the conventional medication's that were being suggested. She agreed to a three-month trial of working on her gut, her mind, and removing toxic people, foods, and situations from her life. I also put her on some key supplements to help reset her brain and calm her nervous system in addition to gut repairing supplements. Three months later, when I saw her for her next hormone appointment, I couldn't believe the shift! I was amazed at how her aura was light and positive, and she was smiling for the first time ever!

I asked her how things were going, and to give me an update. She couldn't believe how much better she felt on all the supplements, but one of the key pieces of advice that she followed was ending some toxic relationships. She and her husband were doing better than ever, were intimate again, and even going on their first vacation together in many years. This is a great example of a patient whose hormones had been optimized for several years, but she was still missing some key pieces to help her feel whole and at peace- mind, body, and spirit.

Toxic people, thoughts and thinking can harm us in several ways, both mentally and physically.

Here are some of the ways toxic thoughts can have a negative impact on our well-being:

1. **Increased stress:** Toxic thoughts often revolve around negativity, self-doubt, worry, or anger. Continuous engagement with such thoughts triggers the body's stress response, leading to the release of stress hormones like cortisol. Prolonged exposure to high levels of stress hormones can have detrimental effects on our physical and mental health, including weakened immune system, sleep disturbances, and increased risk of anxiety and depression.

"Toxic people, thoughts and thinking can harm us in several ways, both mentally and physically."

2. **Impaired mental health:** Toxic thoughts can contribute to the development or exacerbation of mental health conditions such as anxiety, depression, and obsessive-compulsive disorder (OCD). Negative thinking patterns can distort our perception of reality, reinforce negative beliefs about ourselves and the world, and hinder our ability to cope with challenges effectively.

3. **Negative self-image:** Toxic thoughts often involve self-criticism, self-blame, and a harsh inner dialogue. Over time, this can damage our self-esteem and create a negative self-image. Believing negative thoughts about ourselves can impact our confidence, motivation, and overall well-being.

4. **Strained relationships:** Toxic thoughts can influence the way we perceive and interact with others. Negative thinking

patterns, such as constantly assuming the worst intentions of others or holding grudges, can strain relationships and hinder effective communication. It becomes difficult to establish trust and form meaningful connections when our thoughts are clouded by negativity.

5. **Physical health effects:** Research has shown that toxic thoughts and chronic negative emotions can have physical health consequences. Prolonged exposure to negative thinking patterns has been associated with increased risk of cardiovascular problems, compromised immune function, and slower wound healing. Negative thoughts can also impact our behaviors, leading to unhealthy habits such as emotional eating, substance abuse, or a sedentary lifestyle.

6. **Reduced problem-solving skills:** Toxic thoughts tend to be rigid and focused on problems rather than solutions. This can hinder our ability to think creatively, adapt to new situations, and find constructive ways to overcome challenges. It becomes challenging to approach problems with a clear and open mind when our thoughts are clouded by negativity.

It's important to note that occasional negative thoughts are a normal part of life, but it's the persistence and intensity of toxic thoughts that can have a detrimental impact on our well-being. Developing self-awareness, practicing mindfulness, and cultivating positive thinking patterns can help mitigate the harmful effects of toxic thoughts and promote a healthier mindset.

To get a great visual about what negative words we speak over ourselves or from other people can do to our body, search online Dr. Emoto's rice experiment. You will be amazed at what happens to the jars of rice when negative words are spoken towards it. This experiment has been repeated over and over and the results are always the same. The jar of rice that received daily negative statements became molded and rotting, whereas the jar of rice that received positive affirmations remained unchanged. The jar of rice that was completely neglected was somewhere in the middle, with some changes noted in degeneration, but not near to the point of death as the negative jar.

As you can guess, toxic thoughts and relationships can impact gut health. Remember the gut and the brain are interconnected through the gut-brain axis, which allows for communication between the two. This means that what happens in the mind can affect the health of the gut, and vice versa.

"What happens in the mind can affect the health of the gut, and vice versa."

Toxic thoughts and chronic stress can disrupt the balance of the gut microbiota, stress and negative emotions can lead to an imbalance in the gut microbiota composition, reducing the diversity and abundance of beneficial bacteria and promoting the growth of harmful bacteria. This imbalance in the gut microbiota (dysbiosis), can contribute to digestive problems such as irritable bowel syndrome (IBS), inflammatory bowel disease (IBD), and gastrointestinal symptoms like bloating, abdominal pain, and altered bowel movements.

Additionally, chronic stress and negative emotions can affect the movement and contractions of the gastrointestinal tract, leading to symptoms like diarrhea, constipation, or a combination of both. Stress can also increase gut permeability (leaky gut). Remember, this can allow toxins and bacteria to leak into the bloodstream, triggering an immune response and further inflammation.

Moreover, toxic relationships, characterized by negativity, conflict, and lack of support, can contribute to chronic stress and emotional distress. Such relationship dynamics can perpetuate a cycle of stress and negative thinking, which can impact gut health as mentioned earlier.

It's worth noting that the gut-brain connection is complex, and while toxic thoughts and relationships can impact gut health, it's also possible for gut health issues to contribute to mood disturbances and negative thinking patterns. Taking a holistic approach to well-being by addressing both mental health and gut health is essential for overall health and vitality.

HOW CAN I HEAL MY GUT?

First, pay attention! Believe it or not, in a lot of cases, your body is telling you what is happening inside—or at least giving you clues to ask more questions. All too often, people either ignore these clues or become confused and convinced that everything is normal and assume it must be all "in my head." That typically happens after you see one, or maybe several, healthcare providers who have completed a battery of tests and told you they couldn't find anything wrong.

If you are feeling bloated, belch-y, or experiencing digestive issues, especially after meals, your body is trying to tell you something! Sometimes you may notice certain foods make you feel that way and others do not. Pay attention! I know I ignored these signs when I was younger and eating terribly. I noticed I would get a little bit bloated after meals, and I might have some digestive issues, but I chalked it up to stress. As I got older and couldn't enjoy some of my favorite foods any longer, especially spicy foods, I knew something was wrong. If I ate fresh fruits, vegetables, and lean meats, I noticed I didn't have any problems. When I ate bread, pasta, corn chips, and spicy foods, everything went haywire. Intuitively, I stayed away from those foods that caused issues, but I still didn't understand what was going on until I happened upon a lecture at an integrative health conference about the gut. I went on my own journey of healing my gut based on what I had learned, and now I know if I make the decision to eat those inflammatory foods, I'm going to pay the price. Especially if consumed during times of high stress. The inflammation caused by stress hormones, coupled with inflammatory foods, is a double whammy!

"The inflammation caused by stress hormones, coupled with inflammatory foods, is a double whammy!"

Before I get into a discussion about how you can fix an unhealthy gut, let me tell you a story about my patient who has been on hormone therapy for many years. Over a four year period, she complained of more and more weight gain, stomach pain, bloating, and myriad of digestive issues, as well as a recent onset of joint pain and extreme fatigue. She was convinced she was burning through her hormones too fast and needed a higher dose. She had been to her primary care doctor, who did an exam and referred her to a GI doctor, who put her through a gamut of tests, only to tell her everything was normal. She had tried multiple diets for weight loss, to no avail. She was always bloated, always in pain after every meal, and just kept gaining weight. I told her I thought all her symptoms were related to leaky gut and the pain she was having in her stomach after she ate was not normal. I encouraged her to get a leaky gut blood panel, which tests for antibodies that are produced when you have intestinal permeability issues. It also tests for Celiac disease and gluten intolerances. Two weeks later, when I got her results back, I was not surprised that she had a leaky gut and gluten sensitivity, but I was surprised she had Celiac disease.

Celiac disease is an autoimmune disorder in which the body's immune system reacts to gluten; as you probably know, gluten is a protein found in wheat, barley, and rye. When people with Celiac disease consume gluten, their immune system mistakenly attacks the lining of the small intestine, causing inflammation and damage to the villi - small, finger-like projections that line the small intestine and absorb nutrients from food. Over time, the damage to the villi can lead to malabsorption of important nutrients, such as iron, calcium, and vitamin D, which can lead to a range of health problems. Symptoms of Celiac disease can vary widely and may include gastrointestinal symptoms, such as abdominal pain, bloating, and diarrhea, as well as non-gastrointestinal symptoms, such as fatigue, anemia, and joint pain, all of which this patient had.

I told her she needed to immediately get off gluten, start on an anti-inflammatory diet, and begin the process of healing her leaky gut with certain supplements and foods. She took the blood test back to her G.I. doctor, who promptly told her, "There's no way to diagnose Celiac through a blood test; the only way to diagnose Celiac is through a biopsy of the small intestine." So, he scheduled her to do the procedure the following day. A week later, I got a message from her hospital bed that when the G.I. doctor went into her small intestine with the scope to get a biopsy, he punctured her bowel because her small intestine was so thin and inflamed from the severity of her Celiac disease. She was in the ICU for over a week! She was very upset that her G.I. doctor did not correlate the lab test with presentation of symptoms and make the logical diagnosis. Instead, he allowed his confirmation bias to make the diagnosis and it almost cost her life .

For this patient, like many others, the signs of gluten sensitivity and gluten allergies were present long before it led to celiac disease, but unfortunately, many of those warning signs are ignored or blown off, usually by healthcare providers, until it's too late. This type of story, although maybe not as dramatic of an outcome as my patient, is not uncommon. What is so obvious to those of who understand the gut and how vital good gut health is, and what an unhealthy gut can manifest as, is all too often not recognized, and sometimes ignored, by many Western doctors. Again, usually, this is no fault of their own; it is just not how they were trained. It's just not how I was trained! I never received any education about the gut microbiome or leaky gut in my basic clinical training.

Goodbye, dysbiosis; hello, eubiosis!

Eubiosis refers to a state of balanced and healthy microbial communities. In eubiosis, the diversity and composition of the gut microbiota are in a state that supports good health and functioning of the gut and the overall body. Eubiosis is characterized by the presence of a wide variety of beneficial bacteria that work together to support digestion, absorption of nutrients, immune function, and overall health. In a state of eubiosis, these beneficial bacteria can prevent the growth and spread of harmful bacteria and other microorganisms, which can lead to gut dysbiosis and a range of health problems.

Factors that can contribute to eubiosis include a diet rich in fiber and nutrients, regular exercise, adequate sleep, and stress management. On the other hand, factors such as a diet high in processed foods and added sugars, lack of physical activity, inadequate sleep, chronic stress, and certain medications, such as those noted previously, can disrupt the gut microbiome and contribute to dysbiosis. No one wants to hear this! We all want our proverbial (in this case literal) "cake and eat it too". But it does come at a price.

Overall, eubiosis is an important state for maintaining health and wellness, particularly in the gut and immune system, and is a key goal of many interventions aimed at improving gut health. Studies have shown that dietary interventions, such as increasing the intake of fiber and other plant-based foods, probiotic and prebiotic supplementation all can improve the diversity and abundance of beneficial gut bacteria and reduce the risk of inflammatory diseases. Avoiding inflammatory foods, primarily processed foods and sugar being the most inflammatory foods consumed, as well as gluten in many cases, can pave the way for healing a leaky gut.

Recap: strategies to promote eubiosis:

1. **Diet:** A healthy diet is the most important factor for promoting a diverse and balanced gut microbiome. The Mediterranean diet is shown in studies to promote the best health outcomes compared to other diets.

2. **Eating a variety** of fiber-rich fruits and vegetables, whole grains, lean protein, and healthy fats can help nourish

beneficial gut bacteria. It is vital to limit, or eliminate, processed foods, processed sugars, and unhealthy fats (like seed oils), which can promote the growth of harmful gut bacteria as well as contribute to intestinal permeability issues.

3. **Probiotics and prebiotics:** Probiotics are beneficial bacteria that can be taken as supplements or obtained through fermented foods like yogurt, kefir, and kimchi. Prebiotics are types of fiber that feed and support the growth of beneficial gut bacteria. Both probiotics and prebiotics can help restore a healthy gut microbiome.

4. **Stress reduction:** Stress-reducing activities, such as meditation, yoga, and exercise, can help promote a healthy gut microbiome and heart a leaky gut.

Other lifestyle factors: Adequate sleep, regular exercise, avoiding smoking and excessive alcohol intake can all contribute to a healthy gut microbiome.

STRATEGIES TO HEAL A LEAKY GUT

Let's go back to the young girl I told you about at the beginning of this chapter. Even though she tried to fix her gut by adopting better, dietary habits, she still had problems. That is because her leaky gut was allowing proteins from the healthy foods to "leak" into her bloodstream and continue the inflammatory process. She did the right thing by changing her diet, but what was missing was everything she needed to heal and repair those tight junctions in her gut lining. Repairing a leaky gut is simple, but not always easy, and it takes time. Most people become impatient with the time it takes to heal the gut, but one thing you must remember is a leaky gut is usually a process that happens slowly and quietly over several years of poor dietary habits and chronic stress. Unless it is related to a traumatic brain injury, which I said earlier can contribute to a leaky gut within 20 minutes, a leaky gut just doesn't happen overnight.

Once you begin to repair those leaky junctions in the gut wall, it can take up to 12 weeks before you may begin to reintroduce certain foods that caused issues back into your diet. It is important to understand as you start to heal and remove the offending foods from your diet, if you begin to eat them again before your gut is completely healed, you can have a massive histamine response and the misery you felt before you started healing can be 10 times worse!

STEPS TO HEAL A LEAKY GUT:

Step 1: Remove inflammatory foods from your diet.

I have already mentioned these before, and the task can be daunting, but if you start with simply removing anything that comes in a package, you will be well on your way to restoring those tight junctions in your gut. *If you can't pick it, pull it, or kill it, you should not eat it.* In other words, if it doesn't come from a tree, the ground, the land, or the sea (meat, fish, or poultry), you probably should not eat it. I had a patient ask me if it counted if he "pulled" the bag of potato chips out of the pantry—of course not! He knew I meant anything that can be pulled from a tree, like fresh fruit .

Other things that can be inflammatory until your gut heals are some dairy products that contain casein. If you are going to eat dairy products, and you just can't stand the thought of giving up cheese, make sure you are eating European cheeses or butters made from European cows, as they do not have some of the inflammatory proteins of American dairy cows, like casein. Other foods that can be inflammatory to a leaky gut, until it is healed, are nightshade vegetables. Nightshade vegetables include peppers, eggplant, tomatoes, many other beloved vegetables! And it is not that these things are unhealthy, per se, but when you already have a leaky gut, this classification of foods can exacerbate the inflammation and make it difficult, if not impossible, to heal. Moreover, when proteins from those foods get into the bloodstream, the body will create antibodies against those food proteins and recognize them as foreign, so every time you eat them, if your gut is not repaired, you will experience a worsening immune response.

Additional things that can be very inflammatory and impede healing of your gut is chronic alcohol intake, especially wines that are highly processed with sugars and not organic! I will take a moment to talk about organic foods, but often, many people don't consider wine a problem. Red wine is good for you, right? Resveratrol is one of many health benefits of wine, but many American wineries use pesticides on their grapes and speed up the fermentation process by adding sugar, both of which can produce a very inflammatory product. If you are a wine lover like I am, I recommend you stick to organic or European wines, as they are naturally organic (no pesticides allowed!), are drier, and are known as biologic wines, meaning they make their wines in the old way, slow and steady without adding or using chemicals to speed the process or increase the crop yield. There are many wineries in US that have re-adopted the old processes of winemaking and attempt to eliminate pesticides and other chemicals from their grape-growing process.

The reason organic foods and wines are so much more preferred is they have not been intentionally sprayed with pesticides such as glysphosphate. Glysphosphate is a known chemical that is a direct cause of leaky gut; you probably know it as the pesticide spray marketed as Round-up. Glysphosphate has been banned in many countries, as have genetically modified (GMO) foods, because of the known harmful effects on human and animal health. Sadly, not in the United States, where it is still widely used in our commercial farming industries. More on commercially farmed and raised foods in the next chapter.

Finally, don't discount the inflammatory role that chronic stress plays in your life. Now, I know there are many stressors that cannot be avoided, like work stress and general everyday stress of life, but there are things you can do to mitigate the stress in your life. Number one, put down the phone, close the computer, and turn off other electronics! The constant light from electronic devices and the stress on the brain from continual sensory stimulus and chronic bad news and negative information found on social and news media platforms have been known to keep cortisol levels elevated. Cortisol is a key player in inflammation and gut health.

Exercise, meditation, doing things that bring you a sense of peace—whether that is engaging in spiritual practices, prayer, spending time with friends who are positive and uplifting, taking a nice walk in the evenings, deep breathing, yoga—whatever it is that brings you a sense of calm, you need to do, and often!

That may mean removing toxic, stressful people from your life! You know who they are; remove them, or yourself from them, as best as you can.

I had a patient who couldn't figure out why she always felt so sick to her stomach and bloated after eating. She lived a life of extreme stress as a single working mom trying to make ends meet after getting out of a very toxic and abusive marriage. She had done everything she knew to adopt a healthy lifestyle. Besides eliminating toxic, abusive people from her life, she eliminated all processed foods and adopted a healthier lifestyle of exercise and increasing fresh fruits and vegetables. When I dug into the foods she was eating every day, the biggest offender in her diet at that time was the beautiful ripe tomatoes she was growing in her garden; she ate them with every single meal. She was very sad to hear that until her leaky gut was repaired, she was going to have to give up the tomatoes, but when she stopped eating them her pain, bloating and gas went away. She started the steps to repair her leaky gut, and the following year, when tomatoes were back in season, she happily reported she could eat her prized tomatoes again without any issues.

Step 2: Repair your leaky gut with healing foods and key nutrients known to close the leaky junctions:

1. **Fermented foods:** Fermented foods such as kimchi, sauerkraut, kefir, and yogurt contain beneficial probiotic bacteria that can help to improve gut health.

2. **Bone broth:** Bone broth is rich in collagen, which is a type of protein that can help to repair and strengthen the gut lining.

3. **Non-starchy vegetables:** Non-starchy vegetables such as broccoli, cauliflower, kale, and spinach are high in fiber and nutrients that can support healthy gut bacteria and reduce inflammation.

4. **Healthy fats:** Healthy fats such as those found in avocados, nuts, seeds, and fatty fish like salmon can help to reduce inflammation and promote gut health.

5. **Prebiotic foods:** Prebiotic foods such as garlic, onions, and asparagus contain fiber that can help to feed beneficial gut bacteria. Natural fiber is also pre-biotic.

6. **Probiotics:** Probiotics are beneficial bacteria that can help to improve gut health and reduce inflammation. Taking a high-quality probiotic supplement may be beneficial for those with a leaky gut.

7. **Glutamine:** Glutamine is an amino acid that is essential for maintaining the integrity of the gut lining. Supplementation with glutamine helps to reduce inflammation and promote gut healing. When healing a leaky gut, you will need at least 5 g, or 5000 mg, of glutamine daily.

8. **Zinc:** Zinc is a mineral that plays a role in immune function and gut health. Supplementation with zinc may help to reduce inflammation and improve gut permeability.

9. **Cats claw:** Cats claw is plant that has several beneficial properties, such as antioxidant, anti-inflammatory, antimicrobial, as well as protecting the gut barrier and promoting the production of mucus, reducing gut permeability.

10. **Vitamin D:** Vitamin D is a nutrient that is important for immune function and may also play a role in gut health. Supplementation with vitamin D may be beneficial for those with a leaky gut.

11. **Omega-3 fatty acids:** Omega-3 fatty acids are healthy fats that have anti-inflammatory properties. Supplementation with omega-3s may help to reduce inflammation and promote gut health.

Again, the steps are simple, but often not easy, especially the part about removing toxic people from your life. However, once you begin the process of healing, you'll realize when you let those toxic foods, habits, and people back into your life, even just for a day, you can go backwards quickly! I have had some people argue that all this healthy organic eating is more expensive! Well, when you add up the expenses of managing chronic diseases like cancer, heart, disease, diabetes, and chronic pain, not to mention the expense of lost income from time away from work, the expense of an unhealthy lifestyle is much greater than the expense of buying and preparing organic, fresh meats, fruits, and vegetables. The time and other resources spent giving care to your body in this way will pay dividends in the long run .

CHAPTER 10

NUTRITION & HORMONE HEALTH

"In the 21st century our taste buds, our brain chemistry, our biochemistry, our hormones and our kitchens have been hijacked by the food industry."
Mark Hyman, MD

"Let food be thy medicine and thy medicine be thy food."
Hippocrates

Many people have asked if consuming organic, pasture-raised meat, poultry, and eggs, versus commercially raised poultry and eggs, and grass-fed and finished beef, as opposed to commercially prepared beef, is a worthy investment. I would say absolutely, yes. The research is finally coming around to show that feeding animals a diet of GMO corn and other grains, as well as the stress of crowded and confined spaces, antibiotic, and hormone use, all create inflammatory hormones in the animal. When the animals are prepared for consumption, those inflammatory hormones are passed on to whoever eats that animal. Animals in the wild do not eat corn and grain; they are also free to roam and not crowded together in pens or stalls.

Cows eat grass, and chickens eat bugs! Feeding these animals anything outside what is natural for them to consume and raising them anywhere outside their natural habitat can only cause disastrous effects on the health of not only the animals, but also those who consume them.

The food supply in the US is facing a mineral and nutrient crisis. There are several factors that can contribute to a potential decline in the nutrient content of food, including:

1. **Soil depletion:** Overuse of soil, as well as the use of chemical fertilizers and pesticides, can lead to soil depletion and a decrease in the nutrient content of the crops grown in that soil.

2. **Modern farming practices:** Many modern farming practices, such as monoculture (growing only one crop in an area), use of genetically modified crops, and the use of chemical fertilizers and pesticides, can lead to a decline in the nutrient content of crops over time.

3. **Food processing:** Many foods that are processed or packaged can lose nutrient content during processing due to exposure to heat, light, and air.

4. **Long transportation times:** Many fruits and vegetables are transported long distances before they reach the consumer, and this can result in a loss of nutrient content and taste.

5. **Breeding for yield and appearance:** Crops are often bred for maximum yield and appearance, which can lead to a decrease in nutrient content and flavor.

Overall, the nutrient content of food farmed in America can vary depending on the specific farming practices, the type of crop, and the processing and transportation methods used. However, research suggests that in some cases, the nutrient content of crops has declined over time due to these factors. *Mass farming of livestock in America has had several impacts on the quality and nutrient content of meat processed in America.* Some of the ways in which this has occurred include:

1. **Diet of the animals:** Many livestock are fed grain-based diets, which can result in a less nutritious meat product than those fed a more natural diet of grasses or forages.

2. **Use of antibiotics and growth hormones:** Many livestock are given antibiotics and growth hormones to promote growth and prevent disease, which can have negative impacts on the quality and nutrient content of the meat.

3. **Stressful living conditions:** The crowded living conditions of many livestock in mass-farming operations can lead to increased stress, which can have negative impacts on the quality of the meat.

4. **Processing methods:** The processing of meat in large-scale facilities can result in a loss of nutrient content due to exposure to heat and other processing methods.

5. **Additives and preservatives:** Many processed meats contain additives and preservatives, which can have negative impacts on the nutrient content of the meat.

As mentioned previously, grass-fed and finished, pasture-raised meats and cage-free chickens and eggs that are also pasture raised is key. Of mention, make sure you look for meat that is grass-fed and finished. Some products will market their meats as grass-fed, but that typically means they were fed on grass for a while, but then fattened up on corn and grain before slaughter.

Farm-raised fish can also be a problem for our health. Farm-raised fish can potentially be an unhealthy option due to several factors, including:

1. **Contaminants:** Some farm-raised fish may contain high levels of contaminants such as mercury, polychlorinated biphenyls (PCBs), and dioxins, which can have negative health effects.

2. **Antibiotics and other chemicals:** Like other forms of livestock farming, farm-raised fish may be treated with antibiotics and other chemicals to prevent disease, which can contribute to antibiotic resistance and have negative health effects for consumers.

3. **Nutrient deficiencies:** Some farm-raised fish may have lower levels of omega-3 fatty acids, which are beneficial for heart health and brain function, compared to wild-caught fish.

4. **Environmental impact:** Farm-raised fish can have negative impacts on the environment, such as water pollution and the spread of disease to wild fish populations.

5. **Quality of feed:** The quality of the feed given to farm-raised fish can vary and, in some cases, may not provide the same nutritional value as the natural diets of wild fish.

I have had many patients ask me why they can travel to European countries and eat pasta and bread and never feel bloated or sick. I have experienced the same thing when I was blessed enough to travel to Europe a few years ago. While in Italy, I noticed that eating the pasta and the bread did not make me sick like it did when I eat it in the States. When we traveled to France, I couldn't believe how fruits tasted like the actual fruit! Tomatoes were ripe and juicy and tasted like a tomato! I hadn't tasted fruit and food that fresh and flavorful since I was a kid. Moreover, I slept so great! Even adjusting to the European lifestyle of drinking wine and eating dinners late into the evening I slept well. If I was to eat a meal and drink local wine at 9 o'clock at night back home, I would be awake all night in misery with an inflamed gut.

Why is that? Well, it's because most European countries like France and Italy do not allow glysphosphate and other pesticides sprayed on their crops, everything is essentially organic. Further, they don't mass farm. They also grow in season from smaller local farms rather than mass farming like the states. When you get produce at local farmers markets, you will typically find the freshest available produce because it was picked for ripeness and immediate sale. Most grocery stores in France and Italy stock produce from local farmers. They tend to their soil the way it's meant to be tended to in order to maintain nutrients and produce the best crops.

It is vitally important that the human food supply provides the most nutrition possible for optimal, or at least the best possible, health outcomes. The endocrine disruptors that come from the farming techniques mentioned previously can be a huge problem.

Remember, endocrine disruptors from prior chapters—those sneaky chemicals that get into the body and wreak havoc on your hormone systems? Many of them are quite easily avoidable, and some have already been mentioned.

Here are a few important ways you can avoid endocrine disruptors:

1. **Choose organic foods** - Organic foods are grown without the use of synthetic pesticides and fertilizers, which can contain endocrine-disrupting chemicals.

2. **Use natural personal care products** - Many personal care products, such as lotions, shampoos, and cosmetics, contain chemicals that can disrupt hormones. Look for products that are free of parabens, phthalates, and synthetic fragrances.

3. **Avoid plastic containers** - Many plastics contain endocrine-disrupting chemicals, such as bisphenol A (BPA) and phthalates. Choose glass or stainless-steel containers for food and drinks whenever possible. Especially water bottles!!

4. **Filter your water** - Drinking water can contain endocrine-disrupting chemicals, such as atrazine and perchlorate. Halides are also potentially dangerous- chloride, bromide, and even fluoride found in our drinking water. Use a water filter that is certified to remove these contaminants.

5. **Avoid canned foods** - Many canned foods are lined with BPA, which can leach into the food. Choose fresh or frozen fruits and vegetables instead.

6. **Use natural cleaning products** - Many cleaning products contain chemicals that can disrupt hormones. Look for natural alternatives, such as vinegar, baking soda, and essential oils.

7. **Use fragrance-free products** - Synthetic fragrances can contain endocrine-disrupting chemicals. Choose fragrance-free products whenever possible.

8. **Reduce exposure to pesticides** - Pesticides can contain endocrine-disrupting chemicals. Choose organic produce whenever possible or wash fruits and vegetables thoroughly before eating.

9. **Be mindful of workplace exposure** - Certain jobs, such as those in agriculture, manufacturing, and healthcare, can expose you to endocrine-disrupting chemicals.

Remember, it is impossible to completely avoid exposure to endocrine disruptors, but by being mindful of the products you use and the foods you eat, you can help reduce your exposure and promote a healthier environment.

Lastly, I want to make you aware of the harmful effects of seed oils. Seed oils, known endocrine disruptors, such as soybean, canola, corn, and sunflower oils (to name a few oils made from seeds), are commonly used in processed foods and cooking, but they can be harmful to human health when consumed in excess (think packaged foods, salad dressings, all fast food, etc.) or as a primary source of fat. Instead of seed oils for cooking, use tallow, olive oil, avocado oil or ghee (clarified butter).

Here are some ways that seed oils can be harmful to human health:

1. **Omega-6 to omega-3 imbalance:** Seed oils are high in omega-6 fatty acids, which can promote inflammation in the body when consumed in excess, particularly when there is an imbalance with omega-3 fatty acids. Diets that are high in omega-6 fatty acids and low in omega-3 fatty acids have been linked to an increased risk of chronic diseases, such as heart disease, cancer, and diabetes.

2. **Oxidation and formation of harmful compounds:** Seed oils are high in polyunsaturated fats, which are more prone to oxidation than saturated or monounsaturated fats. Oxidation can lead to the formation of harmful compounds, such as free radicals and advanced glycation end products (AGEs), which can contribute to inflammation and other negative health effects.

3. **Processing and refining:** Many seed oils are heavily processed and refined, which can result in the loss of important nutrients and the formation of harmful compounds, such as trans fats.

4. **Potential contaminants:** Some seed oils may contain trace amounts of pesticides, solvents, or other contaminants, which can be harmful to human health if consumed in high amounts.

NUTRACEUTICALS

A patient of mine asked one day if I would see her 18-year-old son. She was concerned about him because over the prior 3 years he had been placed on ADD medication for focus issues, an antidepressant and sometimes needed a medication for anxiety. She was reading information in my office about testosterone decline in men and realized her son had almost all the symptoms. I agreed to see him. Prior to going into the room for his visit, I looked over his labs and was surprised to see his testosterone level was over 900. His vitamin D was low, his B 12 was low as was his iodine.

Sadly, in Texas we see a lot of steroid abuse among high school football players trying to get bigger. Often their own fathers are helping them find these medications on the internet. What they don't realize, and I have seen this all too often, is anabolic steroid use can permanently shut down testosterone production, leading to infertility, and all of the other life altering symptoms of testosterone deficiency. Based on the mom's description of his issues, I fully expected to walk into the room of buffed out football player, but to my surprise, this was a tall, lanky normal teenager. After an exam and review of his health and diet history, which was terrible as you can imagine, I addressed his nutritional deficiencies with education about his diet and placed him on vitamin D3, B complex and iodine.

In two months when I next saw his mom for hormone treatment, she said "I just want to thank you, you saved my kids life! I couldn't get him to take a chewable vitamin as a kid, but now he is calling me from college asking me to send him more supplements! And", she said, "he is off all of his medications!" You see he had fuel in the tank, but he lacked the nutritional support to get that fuel into the engine to do the work.

In addition to the key supplements to promote a healthy gut that I spoke of in the previous chapter, there are other key nutraceuticals that play an active role in optimizing hormone levels, as well as hormone receptor activity. A nutraceutical is a type of dietary supplement or functional food that contains bioactive compounds (meaning they influence the body or cells) derived from natural sources, such as plants, herbs, and foods. They come in various forms for use, like vitamins, minerals, antioxidants, prebiotics, probiotics, herbal extracts, and other natural compounds. Many are believed to have health benefits and can be used to support overall health, prevent chronic disease, and improve certain health conditions. Nutraceuticals are not regulated by the FDA in the same way that prescription drugs are, and their efficacy and safety may vary depending on the specific product and its source. In fact, one study showed that up to 70 percent of the nutrition supplements on the market in the US either don't have the stated ingredients on the label and/or contain harmful contaminants of some kind. This is why it is so important to purchase pharmaceutical-grade nutraceuticals.

"One study showed that up to 70 percent of the nutrition supplements on the market in the US either don't have the stated ingredients on the label and/or contain harmful contaminants of some kind."

Before I get into a discussion about some key nutraceuticals that support hormone therapy, I want to tell you a story about a patient who has been on hormone pellet therapy for many years. She came for an appointment to get her next hormone pellet insertion, and when I asked her how she was doing, she stated, "I don't think these hormone pellets are working anymore." I asked her what she meant, and she said she just didn't feel the same as she did when she first started, and she was not sure why. I asked her if she was still taking the supplements I prescribed at the beginning of our time together. She said she stopped taking all her supplements because she was tired of taking them. Knowing how vital D3 is for hormone receptor activity and other actions of hormones in the body, I told her, "Let's make a deal." I said, "Start taking at least your vitamin D between now and our next visit in four months, and if you don't feel a significant improvement, I will refund your money." She looked at me with great surprise and said, "You've got a deal!" Fast forward four months to her next visit, before The appointment began, she said, "I almost don't want to tell you the truth, because I'd love to have my money back, but I will never stop taking my vitamin D again. I can't believe how much better I felt on it."

Remember my analogy earlier in this book regarding having fuel in your gas tank, but it not being able to get into the engine to do its work? These stories are perfect examples; both the 18-year-old male and this patient had hormones, a.k.a. fuel, circulating in the body, but due to nutrient deficiencies, they just couldn't transfer the hormone "fuel" into the cell to exert their actions.

There are many other nutrients that help our body run efficiently the same way. For instance, you need a ferritin level of greater than 70 to convert your thyroid hormone T4 to the active thyroid T3. Selenium plays a role in thyroid function, as well as zinc; there are so many nutrients that, unfortunately, most people are quite deficient in in this country because of the SAD (standard American diet) as well as the quality of our farmed food.

VITAMIN D

Vitamin D, also known as the "sunshine vitamin," is a fat-soluble vitamin that is essential for overall health. It plays a crucial role in the absorption of calcium and phosphorus, which are important for the development and maintenance of strong bones and teeth. Vitamin D also helps regulate the immune system, supports cardiovascular health, and plays a role in preventing certain types of cancer.

The primary source of vitamin D is exposure to sunlight, which triggers the skin to produce vitamin D3. However, it can also be obtained through the diet, including fatty (wild caught) fish (such as salmon, tuna, and mackerel), fortified dairy products, and supplements. Vitamin D deficiency is a common issue, particularly in people who live in areas with limited sunlight exposure, wear clothing that covers most of the skin, are of dark-skinned ethnicities, or have a diet lacking in vitamin D-rich foods. Dark skinned ethnicities have a natural, built in sunscreen via a higher number of melanocytes, the cells that cause darker skin pigment; but when it comes to D3 absorption, it also blocks this vital nutrient. A deficiency in vitamin D can lead to a variety of health problems, including osteoporosis, increased risk of falls and fractures, increased risk of infections, and autoimmune disorders such as multiple sclerosis.

Research has also suggested that vitamin D deficiency may be also linked to an increased risk of certain types of cancer, including colon, breast, and prostate cancer. Additionally, low vitamin D levels have been associated with an increased risk of cardiovascular disease, including hypertension and heart disease.

To ensure adequate levels of vitamin D, it is recommended adults get at least 5000 IU per day, and children get 2000 iu per day. However, some people may require higher doses to maintain optimal levels (over 60). Supplementation can be helpful for those who are unable to get enough vitamin D through their diet or sun exposure. Special attention should be paid to children, they spend a great deal of time indoors and when they are outdoors, if they are lighter skinned, they are lathered in sunscreen which blocks much of the vitamin d absorption form the sun.

Of course, the best way to get D3 is from sun exposure, without sunscreen of course. Just 20 minutes in the sun between 12-2 may provide up to 20,000 iu of D3!

VITAMIN D & HORMONES

Vitamin D plays a critical role in regulating hormones in the body. It interacts with cells in the endocrine system, which includes the glands that produce hormones, such as the thyroid, parathyroid, and adrenal glands and, like I said earlier, turns on many hormone receptors!

"Vitamin D plays a critical role in regulating hormones in the body."

One of the primary functions of vitamin D in the endocrine system is its role in regulating the production of parathyroid hormone (PTH). PTH is produced by the parathyroid glands and helps regulate calcium and phosphorus levels in the blood. When calcium levels in the blood drop, PTH is released, and it helps increase calcium levels by releasing calcium from the bones and increasing absorption in the intestines. Vitamin D helps regulate PTH production by increasing calcium absorption in the intestines, which helps reduce the need for PTH release.

In addition to regulating PTH, vitamin D also plays a role in regulating the production of other hormones, such as insulin and testosterone. Studies have found that vitamin D deficiency is associated with an increased risk of insulin resistance and type-II diabetes, possibly due to the role that vitamin D plays in insulin production and sensitivity. Similarly, vitamin D is also involved in the production and regulation of testosterone. Overall, vitamin D is a critical component in the endocrine system, and its role in regulating hormone production and function is essential for overall health and wellbeing.

VITAMIN D AND CHRONIC METABOLIC DISEASES

Vitamin D has been linked to the prevention and management of chronic diseases, including cardiovascular disease. Several studies have found that low levels of vitamin D are associated with an increased risk of cardiovascular disease, such as heart attack, stroke, and heart failure. One of the ways in which vitamin D may reduce the risk of cardiovascular disease is through its role in regulating blood pressure. Vitamin D helps to reduce the levels of renin, an enzyme that increases blood pressure by constricting blood vessels. By reducing renin levels, vitamin D can help to lower blood pressure and reduce the risk of developing hypertension, a major risk factor for cardiovascular disease.

Another way in which vitamin D may reduce the risk of cardiovascular disease is through its anti-inflammatory properties. As you have learned, chronic inflammation is a contributing factor to the development of cardiovascular disease, and studies have shown that vitamin D can help to reduce inflammation in the body. Vitamin D may also improve endothelial function, which is the ability of blood vessels to relax and expand in response to increased blood flow. Impaired endothelial function is a precursor to atherosclerosis, the buildup of plaque in the arteries that can lead to heart attack and stroke. Vitamin D has been shown to improve endothelial function and reduce the risk of atherosclerosis.

Furthermore, vitamin D can also help to reduce the risk of diabetes, a significant risk factor for cardiovascular disease. Vitamin D plays a role in insulin secretion and sensitivity, and low levels of vitamin D have been associated with an increased risk of insulin resistance and type-II diabetes. Overall, vitamin D plays a crucial role in reducing the risk of several chronic diseases through its effects on blood pressure, inflammation, endothelial function, and insulin sensitivity.

VITAMIN D & CANCER

There is evidence to suggest that vitamin D may play a role in the prevention and management of certain cancers. Studies have shown that low blood levels of vitamin D (under 60) are associated with an increased risk of several types of cancer, including breast, colon, prostate, and pancreatic cancer. One way in which vitamin D may reduce the risk of cancer is through its ability to regulate cell growth and division. Vitamin D helps to control the expression of genes that are involved in cell proliferation, differentiation, and apoptosis (cell death). Abnormal cell growth and division can lead to the development of cancer, and vitamin D may help to prevent this by regulating cell growth.

"Blood levels of vitamin D (under 60) are associated with an increased risk of several types of cancer, including breast, colon, prostate, and pancreatic cancer."

Additionally, vitamin D has anti-inflammatory properties that may help to reduce the risk of cancer. Chronic inflammation is also a risk factor for cancer, and vitamin D has been shown to reduce inflammation in the body. Furthermore, vitamin D may help to boost the immune system's ability to fight cancer. Vitamin D has been shown to enhance the function of immune cells, such as T cells and natural-killer cells, which play a crucial role in identifying and destroying cancer cells. Studies have also found that vitamin D may help to reduce the risk of cancer metastasis, which is the spread of cancer cells to other parts of the body. Vitamin D has been shown to inhibit the growth and migration of cancer cells and may help to prevent the spread of cancer to other organs.

VITAMIN K2

Vitamin K2 is a type of vitamin K that is important for bone and cardiovascular health. It works by activating proteins that help to regulate calcium metabolism in the body. One of the main roles of vitamin K2 is its ability to activate a protein called osteocalcin. Osteocalcin is produced by bone cells and helps to regulate bone formation and mineralization. Vitamin K2 activates osteocalcin by adding a chemical group called a gamma-carboxyl group to the protein, which allows it to bind to calcium and other minerals in the bones. Vitamin K2 also activates another protein called matrix Gla protein (MGP), which is important for preventing the buildup of calcium in blood vessels. MGP helps to regulate the transport of calcium from the blood vessels to the bones and other tissues, preventing the buildup of calcium in the arteries that can lead to cardiovascular disease.

The relationship between vitamin K2 and vitamin D is important for overall health. Vitamin D helps to increase calcium absorption from the diet and helps to maintain calcium levels in the blood. However, without adequate vitamin K2, calcium may be deposited in soft tissues, such as blood vessels, rather than in the bones and teeth where it is needed. Research suggests that vitamin K2 may help to improve the balance between vitamin D and calcium in the body. By activating osteocalcin and MGP, vitamin K2 helps to ensure that calcium is properly absorbed and utilized by the bones and other tissues, reducing the risk of calcium deposition in soft tissues.

WHY A, D, AND K2 TOGETHER?

Overall, taking vitamin A, vitamin D, and vitamin K2 together can help to support bone health, immune function, and cardiovascular health. Vitamin A is a fat-soluble vitamin that is important for a variety of functions in the body. It is essential for maintaining healthy vision, immune function, and skin health, as well as playing a role in growth and development. Vitamin A works together with vitamin D and vitamin K2 to support bone health. Recall, vitamin D helps to increase the absorption and utilization of calcium in the body, while vitamin K2 helps to ensure that calcium is properly deposited in the bones and not in soft tissues. Vitamin A plays a role in bone health by regulating the activity of osteoclasts, cells that break down and remodel bone tissue.

In addition, vitamin A is important for immune function, and it works together with vitamin D to support the immune system. Vitamin A is essential for the development and maintenance of mucosal surfaces, such as those in the respiratory and digestive tracts, which act as barriers to infection. Vitamin D helps to regulate the activity of immune cells, including those that help to fight off infection. Vitamin A also plays a role in skin health, as it is essential for the growth and maintenance of skin cells. It can help to prevent and treat skin conditions such as acne, psoriasis, and eczema.

HOW MUCH A, D, & K IS OPTIMAL?

Optimal vitamin D levels are greater than 60, even though 30-100 is considered the "reference range." Remember that right side of the bell curve average? Vitamin D is one of those blood reference ranges that you want to have on the right side of the curve for all the benefits discussed previously. Studies have found it takes 5000 IU daily for adults to keep their levels in the optimal range. For darker skin ethnicities, that is probably going to be higher because darker skin ethnicities do not absorb vitamin D through the skin from the sun as lighter skinned people do.

A general rule of thumb in my clinical practice that I have seen help get the levels in optimal range is 10,000 IUs a day if blood levels of D3 are under 30 and 5000 IUs a day if levels are greater than 30. The vitamin D council has recommended that children get a minimum of 2000 IU of vitamin D a day, especially darker skin ethnicities.

How much K2 is optimal? The jury still out on that, but what is known is that it takes at least 500 μg (micrograms) of vitamin K2 to activate the body's K2-dependent proteins and elicit all the actions that have been discussed. Optimal vitamin A intake should be close to the same amount as your vitamin D to work synergistically with D3. For instance, if you're taking 5000 IU D3, you should have a supplement that has 5000 IU of vitamin A.

Of mention, there is some old information out there that has frightened some people away from vitamin D and vitamin A because of concerns of toxicity. Understand many old recommendations are based on very bad clinical studies. In all the studies that presumed vitamin D3 was toxic, it wasn't the D3; it was the calcium. Remember, when you raise your D3, you increase your calcium absorption and levels. If you don't have the other nutrients to help shuttle calcium where it belongs or excrete excess calcium out of the kidneys, you certainly can become "toxic" or have a problem called hypercalcemia, which basically means too much calcium. High calcium levels can cause muscle twitching and other vague symptoms, so it is important to have your calcium levels checked periodically if you are taking higher doses of vitamin D, especially without the supporting nutrients of A and K2.

In one very poor study on vitamin A, they concluded that vitamin a can be toxic. In this study, however, they were giving patients 100,000 IU a day of vitamin A! That is ridiculously high and so far off the recommended doses, so of course they would have problems! Vitamin A can be toxic to the liver and cause other issues, but usually only when taking for a long period of time and extremely high doses, not in the ranges recommended to support calcium excretion with D3 and K2.

SUPPLEMENTS TO HELP OPTIMIZE HORMONE HEALTH AND METABOLISM

There are several other nutrient supplements that can aid in proper hormone metabolism, including:

1. **Magnesium:** Magnesium plays a critical role in hormone regulation, including the production of estrogen, progesterone, and testosterone. It can help to alleviate symptoms of PMS and menopause, and it can also support adrenal function and reduce stress levels.

2. **Zinc:** Zinc is essential for proper hormone production and metabolism, particularly for testosterone and thyroid hormones. It can also help to balance estrogen levels and improve insulin sensitivity.

3. **Vitamin D:** Vitamin D is important to produce hormones, including testosterone and estrogen. It can also help to regulate the menstrual cycle and reduce symptoms of PMS.

4. **B vitamins:** B vitamins, particularly vitamin B6, are important for hormone regulation, including the production of estrogen and progesterone. They can also help to reduce stress levels and support adrenal function.

5. **Omega-3 fatty acids:** Omega-3 fatty acids can help to reduce inflammation in the body, which can improve hormone balance. They can also help to support adrenal function and reduce stress levels.

6. **Adaptogenic herbs:** Adaptogenic herbs such as ashwagandha, rhodiola, and holy basil can help to regulate cortisol levels and reduce stress levels. They can also support adrenal function and improve hormone balance.

KEY NUTRACEUTICALS FOR OPTIMAL THYROID FUNCTION

The thyroid gland requires several nutrients to produce, convert, and regulate thyroid hormones. Below are some beneficial nutrients to aid in thyroid hormone metabolism:

1. **Iodine:** Iodine is a critical component of thyroid hormones. The body cannot produce iodine on its

own, so it is important to consume iodine-rich foods such as seaweed, fish, dairy, and eggs. In some cases, supplementation may be necessary.

2. **Selenium:** Selenium is an important mineral for thyroid function, as it helps to convert inactive thyroid hormone (T4) to active thyroid hormone (T3). Selenium can be found in Brazil nuts, seafood, meat, and whole grains. The thyroid gland is particularly rich in selenium, and in individuals with Hashimoto's, selenium supplementation has been shown to have beneficial effects. Studies have also suggested that selenium supplementation may reduce thyroid peroxidase antibodies, which are elevated in Hashimoto's disease and associated with thyroid gland damage. Additionally, selenium appears to have antioxidant effects, which can help to protect the thyroid gland from oxidative stress and inflammation.

3. **Zinc:** Zinc is essential to produce thyroid hormones, and it also helps to convert T4 to T3. Zinc can be found in oysters, beef, pork, chicken, and legumes.

4. **Iron:** Iron is important for thyroid function, as it helps to transport thyroid hormones throughout the body. Iron can be found in red meat, poultry, seafood, beans, and leafy green vegetables.

5. **Vitamin D:** Vitamin D is important for thyroid function, as it helps to regulate the production of thyroid hormones. Vitamin D can be obtained through sun exposure, as well as through fortified foods and supplements.

6. **B vitamins:** B vitamins, particularly vitamin B12, are important for thyroid function. They can be found in meat, fish, dairy, and fortified cereals.

Iodine is worthy of a bit more mention. Iodine is an essential micronutrient used by every single cell in the human body. It was considered the universal medicine from the late 1800s until about 1960s and treated everything! Conditions like goiter, atherosclerosis (a.k.a. hardening of the arteries), sexually transmitted disease, uterine fibroids, prostate enlargement, obesity, depression, breast issues, skin conditions, and so many more! All of our glandular organs have an affinity for iodine, organs like prostate, ovaries, breast, and most notably the thyroid. Seventy to 80% of our iodine is contained in the thyroid! So, you can imagine if you're iodine deficient, none of those organs that need it so desperately can get it because the thyroid is going to take everything! It is required for the synthesis of thyroid hormones, as the thyroid gland uses iodine to produce the hormones thyroxine (T4) and triiodothyronine (T3), which as you now know regulate the body's metabolism, body temperature, heart rate, and other vital functions.

When taking enough iodine, or getting enough through the diet, it neutralizes, cancer- causing cells, can remove abnormal cells, kills viruses, and can neutralize toxins from other microorganisms like bacteria. Iodine has been shown to reverse fibrocystic breast disease, a known risk factor for breast cancer. Iodine deficiency is a significant global health problem and can result in a range of health issues, including goiter (an enlargement of the thyroid gland), hypothyroidism (an underactive thyroid gland), cognitive impairment, and cretinism (a severe form of mental and physical impairment). Iodine deficiency is particularly harmful during pregnancy and early childhood, as it can lead to stunted growth, cognitive impairment, and even stillbirth or miscarriage. One of the primary reasons Americans are so iodine deplete is the lack of minerals in our soil, decreasing the nutrient continent of our soil of vital minerals, including iodine. Another reason is in the 1970s, commercially prepared baked goods, which fortified their products with iodine, began to use a toxic chemical instead called bromide.

There are several great resources and books available about how important iodine is to human health and why it's so important to supplement with iodine. Dr. David Brownstein has done a great deal of work, as well as Dr. David Derry's work on breast cancer and iodine, and a host of others. The recommendations that come from any of these physicians is to get enough iodine that closely mirrors the iron intake of Japanese culture. Breast cancer is nearly nonexistent in the Japanese culture, at least in areas of Japan that have not adopted a Western diet. The average Japanese person consuming a typical Japanese diet will, on average, receive 10 mg of iodine a day. That is well above the US RDA for iodine supplementation but understand the US RDA for iodine is a minimum amount, but not it is not the optimal amount required to help prevent the disease processes discussed.

One last thing, you cannot be allergic to mineral iodine. Many people confuse an allergy with shellfish or radioactive iodine used in some diagnostic studies is the same as an iodine allergy. It is not. With a shellfish allergy, that person is reacting to the protein in the shellfish, not the iodine, and of course, allergies to radioactive iodine are a completely different issue. Just understand that if you have these types of allergies, it is perfectly safe for you to take an iodine supplement and consume foods rich in iodine.

DIM (DIINDOLYLMETHANE)

Another key nutraceutical that plays a vital role in hormone optimization is DIM. DIM is found primarily in cruciferous vegetables, but unfortunately, most of us don't eat enough cruciferous vegetables, like broccoli, cabbage, and brussels sprouts in quantities high enough for disease prevention. DIM has been extensively studied in many areas, not the least of which a potential therapeutic drug with antioxidant potential; it can help memory by protecting against oxidative damage and inflammation, and it can protect the cells in the heart against the inflammatory LPS, as you recall, a key root cause of inflammation and chronic diseases.

DIM has been shown to be highly beneficial in preventing breast cancer and has been used as an adjunctive treatment to chemotherapy in breast cancer, as well as prostate cancer. DIM plays a key role in estrogen metabolism by increasing metabolism of estrogen to the 2-hydroxyestrone, or good estrogen, pathway instead of the 16 and 4-hydroxyestrone pathways which, as you may recall, are potentially `more cancer-causing. In one study, they looked at patients who had fibrocystic breast disease and were BRCA positive, and they supplemented with them for one year at 100 mg a day; what they found were these BRCA carriers had a statistically significant decrease in fibrous breast tissue after one year on their MRI. This is great news because fibrocystic breast disease is a risk factor for developing breast cancer. Women with BRCA are at even higher risk than the average female with fibrocystic breast disease, so anything that can be mitigated with key nutrients and supplements is beneficial!

In my clinical practice, not a single female on hormone therapy leaves without a DIM supplement. It is that important for breast cancer protection. Studies show that supplementation with a micronized form of DIM should be 150 mg to 300 mg a day for women and 300 mg to 600 mg a day for men. I can't stress how important this is because if it is not micronized, it will not be absorbed in the gut.

KEY NUTRACEUTICALS FOR STRESS, ANXIETY AND CALMING THE NERVOUS SYSTEM

There are several natural supplements that are commonly used to support a stressed nervous system. These supplements may help promote relaxation, reduce anxiety, and support overall well-being in addition to exercise, meditation, spiritual practices and of course, removing stressors from your life as much as possible. Here are a few examples:

1. **Ashwagandha:** Ashwagandha is an adaptogenic herb that has been traditionally used in Ayurvedic medicine to help the body cope with stress. It may help reduce anxiety, promote a sense of calmness, and support adrenal function.

2. **Rhodiola rosea:** Rhodiola rosea is another adaptogenic herb that has been used to combat stress and fatigue. It may help improve mood, increase energy levels, and enhance mental performance.

3. **Magnesium:** Magnesium is an essential mineral that plays a role in many bodily processes, including the regulation

of the nervous system. It has calming properties and may help reduce anxiety and promote relaxation.

4. **L-theanine:** L-theanine is an amino acid commonly found in green tea. It has been shown to promote relaxation and reduce stress and anxiety without causing drowsiness. It can be taken as a supplement or consumed in the form of green tea. The best supplement I have found is in the form of Suntheanine.

5. **Omega-3 fatty acids:** Omega-3 fatty acids, particularly EPA and DHA, are essential fats that are beneficial for brain health. They have been shown to have anti-inflammatory effects and may help reduce symptoms of anxiety and depression.

6. **B vitamins:** B vitamins, particularly B6, B9 (folate), and B12, are important for the proper functioning of the nervous system. They play a role in the production of neurotransmitters, such as serotonin and dopamine, which are involved in mood regulation. B vitamin supplements or a balanced diet rich in B vitamins can support nervous system health.

There are 2 additional amazing supplements that I have found to be priceless when it comes to stress management: Holy Basil and Relora. Both holy basil (also known as Tulsi) and Relora are natural supplements that are believed to help calm the mind and promote relaxation. In my clinics we use a combination of these plus L-theanine (Suntheanine) called QuiCalm. QuiCalm is one of the top selling supplements in our clinics because it works so well, some patients have said better than Xanax without the drugged feeling!

Here's how they may exert their calming effects:

1. **Holy Basil (Tulsi):** Holy basil is an adaptogenic herb that has been used for centuries in Ayurvedic medicine to support stress management. It is believed to have anxiolytic (anti-anxiety) and antidepressant properties. Holy basil contains compounds like eugenol, rosmarinic acid, and ocimumosides, which may help modulate neurotransmitters and regulate the stress response. It is also known for its antioxidant and anti-inflammatory properties, which can support overall well-being and a healthy nervous system.

2. **Relora:** Relora is a proprietary blend of two plant extracts: Magnolia officinalis and Phellodendron amurense. It is commonly used to help reduce stress, anxiety, and improve mood. Magnolia bark extract in Relora has been found to have anxiolytic effects by interacting with GABA receptors, which are involved in promoting relaxation and reducing anxiety. Phellodendron bark extract in Relora is believed to modulate cortisol levels, a stress hormone that can contribute to anxiety and stress.

It's worth mentioning that supplements alone may not be sufficient to address chronic or severe anxiety or stress. It's important to adopt a holistic approach to stress management, including lifestyle changes, hormone optimization, relaxation techniques, and seeking professional help if needed.

CHAPTER 11

HORMONE REPLACEMENT THERAPY OPTIONS

"Many marriages break up over hormonal imbalance, which is truly sad because it comes from a lack of understanding. When hormones are put back in balance with natural bioidentical hormones, a woman or man resumes their normal life of feeling good and having days filled with quality".
Suzanne Somers

There are several options to consider when embarking on a journey of optimizing your hormones, whether you are male or female. But what are the differences, and which ones are safer? Which ones work better? Which ones are potentially harmful? These are all questions I have been asked over the last decade and a half, not only by my patients but also by the thousands of healthcare providers in the nationwide network I've referenced.

First, there is a huge difference between bioidentical and synthetic hormones. I think I have made those points clear, but it is especially important when you are talking about estrogen and progesterone. Hormones come in several modalities and can be categorized as either bioidentical or synthetic. They come in shots, creams, oral pills, and capsules, rapid-dissolve tablets (RDT or ODT), and my favorite, bioidentical hormone pellets, that are placed in the fatty tissue under the skin.

I love to give the analogy of a lock and key when I am talking about synthetic versus natural or bioidentical hormones. Have you ever had a key that fits into a lock but doesn't turn the lock and unlock the door? Well, that's very similar to synthetic hormones. They can fit on the receptor "lock," but they don't unlock all the positive benefits as natural hormones do. Bioidentical hormones are like a key that not only fits into the lock but also unlocks the door (to the cell) and allows that hormone to exert its action on the cell in every way it was designed to and without the harmful side effects the synthetic hormones have been shown time and time again to cause. When dosed properly and managed by a healthcare provider who has been extensively trained in the art and science of hormone optimization, hormone therapies can be safe, effective, and used until you are no longer walking the planet!

"When dosed properly and managed by a healthcare provider who has been extensively trained in the art and science of hormone optimization, hormone therapies can be safe, effective, and used until you are no longer walking the planet!"

Like I said, hormone pellet therapy is my favorite option for optimizing hormones for many reasons I will outline shortly. Before I get there, however, I'd like to give you a little bit of background on how I made the leap from traditional modes of hormone replacement therapy to utilizing hormone pellets as the primary mode in my clinical practice. When I first became interested in hormones as a cornerstone of health, most of the trainings I had gone to focused on just estrogen and progesterone for women and testosterone for men. I took what I had learned in several conferences about hormone therapy back to my clinical practice, and I would say I probably helped about 40 percent of the women who came to me. If they were postmenopausal and needed estrogen and progesterone, what I had to offer them worked pretty well. However, there is a large population of my female patients I just couldn't seem to get right. I couldn't seem to address their primary issues of fatigue and weight gain, mood swings, anxiety, depression, and memory loss. The few things I had in my toolbox at the time just weren't cutting it.

About three patients over the span of two weeks called my office to let me know that, regretfully, they were seeing another practitioner who was doing these "testosterone hormone pellets," and it was truly life changing. The last patient I spoke with said, "Dr. Terri, I love you; you're so great to work with, but you need to figure out this testosterone hormone pellet thing." They were talking about a doctor who was using testosterone in his female patients. "Testosterone"? I thought. "What the heck does testosterone have to do with females"? As fate would have it, if you believe in fate, I believe more in divine direction, I connected with this gynecologist, and met to discuss what all this testosterone hormone pellet thing was about.

When he started explaining to me the benefits of testosterone in women and the symptoms that were relieved for his patients, he had only been doing it for a few months at our initial meeting, and all my unanswered questions were answered. All the patients I just couldn't quite get them there, the lightbulb was going off; in fact, the alarm was sounding so loud in my head I asked this physician colleague, "How, when, and where can I get trained on this therapy?" He connected me with a doctor in Scottsdale, Arizona named Gino Tutera. Dr. Tutera had been utilizing hormone pellets in his patients for about 25 years and had been training practitioners in this life-changing therapy. He had learned as a gynecologist about this therapy from his mentor who had been doing pellet therapy for at least 30 years at the time of our meeting in 2009.

I had the honor and privilege to spend an entire day with him in his office; the first half of the day, he reviewed the most up-to-date research studies at the time on the different bioidentical hormones and how pellet therapy works so much better than creams and oral modalities. I was surprised to know that pellet therapy was first being researched in the United States in the 1930s and 40s! I learned that in the 1940s, researchers discovered the female ovary makes testosterones in abundance!

I brought everything that I learned back to Texas and immediately transitioned my hormone therapy patients who were on creams and oral therapies to pellet therapy, including testosterone. The results were astounding. Word of mouth grew my clinical practice at exponential rates, and by December, I had more than quadrupled my patient database. Something else started happening at that time; these women who were suddenly feeling so much better, had their zest for life back, energy and moods were stabilized, and libido came back better than it ever had been, started bringing their husbands in for therapy. Now, the male sector of my practice started growing exponentially, as these guys were sharing with their golf buddies and work colleagues how and why their strength, stamina, mental clarity, and focus, and "pep in their step" had returned. I started getting questions like, "Does testosterone help with joint pain? Does this therapy help decrease belly fat?"

"After about 6-12 months of therapy, having hormones optimized 24/7, I started seeing patients being able to come off their anxiety medications, their antidepressants, their blood pressure medications and oftentimes even type-II diabetes medications."

After about 6-12 months of therapy, having hormones optimized 24/7, I started seeing patients being able to come off their anxiety medications, their antidepressants, their blood pressure medications and oftentimes even type-II diabetes medications. Adult ADD, metabolic syndrome (overweight, high blood pressure, and diabetes), and mood and memory issues were becoming a thing of the past, as I was getting to the root cause of their issues! Not only did I fix many of these issues, but also being able to come off all those medications solved the problems of side effects from those medications and certainly impacted their wallets as well!

I remember thinking after about nine months of using this therapy myself and on my patients how blessed I was to have learned about it. I couldn't believe the life changes I was seeing. I remember thinking fifty-five years of the two pioneers of pellet therapy, Dr. Tutera and his mentor, treating patients in their little corner of the world, changing so many lives; the world needs to know about this therapy! I started doing patient education seminars in the waiting room of my office and speaking at rotary clubs, women's clubs, chamber events, and anywhere I could get an audience. I joined my gynecologist colleagues and (my now-husband) Dan DeNeui—who I was divinely seated next to on the plane to Scottsdale to train with Dr. Tutera—in launching a company whose focus was to train other practitioners on this life-changing therapy so they could impact their patients' lives the same way.

"The world needs to know about this therapy!"

I prefer hormone pellets for many reasons, but primarily because it is the only hormone therapy option that most closely resembles what our bodies do naturally, secrete hormones 24 hours a day, seven days a week, and sometimes in surges that relate to activity levels and stress levels. Hormone pellets, after figuring out the dose, which is based on several factors that highly experienced and trained providers understand, are placed under the skin in the fatty tissue either below the belt or above the belt, depending on the patient. Once placed, these hormone pellets go through a process, a very slow dissolution, and hormone levels slowly begin to rise over the course of two to four weeks. Most hormone levels will peak at four to five weeks. Hormone levels typically stay continuous and steady state on average anywhere from three to five months depending on the patient. Once hormone levels start to fall again, the patient may become symptomatic and simply repeats the pellet procedure to get those levels back up.

I like this modality not only because of the bioidentical nature, but patients seem to feel better because they are not having roller-coaster levels like when you take a pill or give yourself a shot. Your body doesn't dump a bolus of hormones into the system that lasts for a few hours and, in the case of shots or patches, maybe a few days. The ovaries and testes (primarily), and the adrenals to some extent, have a slow, steady rate of hormone secretion called a basal rate, with surges and fluctuations that depend on activity, stress (good or bad) and timing in the mental cycle.

I like to give the analogy of licking a lollipop; the faster you lick the lollipop, the faster it dissolves. The same is true for hormone pellets, as they are placed under the skin in the fatty tissue that has quite a bit of blood flow around them. When you're up and about, awake, and active, whether it's exercising or just generally dealing with a busy day, you are "licking the lollipop" faster and will utilize the hormones at a higher rate. When you are asleep at night and everything is slowed down, your heart rate and blood pressure has decreased, and metabolism slows down, you "lick the lollipop" slower.

My next favorite modality of bioidentical hormones after hormone pellets are rapid-dissolve tablets for testosterone and patches for estradiol. At my clinic, I almost always use oral capsules for progesterone because they have a lovely side effect of sleep! I always tell my female patients they double as a free sleeping pill. You may have noticed I'm not a huge fan of hormone creams. That is because, in my experience, I haven't had very many patients get much benefit from their hormone creams; they are messy and must be applied sometimes twice a day to get appreciable levels, and again, it's that roller-coaster effect. Where hormone creams do play a significant role is utilizing estradiol cream in females who can't take estrogen for some reason and have bladder and vaginal symptoms that the creams can relieve in most cases.

Oral pills for bioidentical estrogen and testosterone hormone replacement, except for micronized natural progesterone, are my least favorite modality because they have the highest potential for negative side effects because metabolites form through the liver when taken orally. This is called the "first pass" effect. First-pass metabolism through the liver is what causes most side effects of all oral medications.

Recap: commonly used bio-identical hormone replacement options

1. Testosterone
    - Oral, shots, cream, oral dissolve tablets, pellets
2. Estradiol (17beta)
    - Oral, patch, cream, oral dissolve tablets, pellets
3. Progesterone (micronized)
    - Oral, cream, oral dissolve tablets
4. DHEA
    - Oral compounded or over the counter
5. Melatonin
    - Oral compounded or over the counter
6. Thyroid (desiccated)
    - Oral

SIDE EFFECTS OF SEX HORMONE THERAPIES

"The only difference between medicine and poison is most often the dose."
Dan DeNeui, CEO

Side effects from hormones and hormone therapies have several variables. The type of hormone—is it bioidentical or synthetic; the modality or route of delivery—is it oral, cream, or a patch, injection, or pellets? The patient's individual metabolism plays a role, their health status, their gut status; every person is a unique individual, and although there are common nuisance side effects of testosterone hormone replacement therapy, side effects from hormones vastly differ from patient to patient.

"You cannot conclude the side effects from one type and modality of hormone therapy to be true for all hormones and hormone modalities."

One of the biggest lessons learned, specifically from the Women's Health Initiative trial, is that you cannot conclude the side effects from one type and modality of hormone therapy to be true for all hormones and hormone modalities. The side effects from shots are vastly different than those from pellets. The side effects from synthetic hormones greatly differ from those from bioidentical hormones, and so forth.

When done properly by a highly trained and experienced healthcare provider in this area, side effects are minimal and are typically nuisance side effects that can be reversed by changing the dose of your hormones. In 2022, I collected data from my two hormone clinics in Texas regarding negative outcomes and side effects. Over a 10-year span, from 2012 to 2022, over 40,000 hormone pellet procedures with estrogen and testosterone, either alone or together, were performed in females across the age spectrum and approximately 21,000 male testosterone pellet procedures. In 2022 alone, our clinics performed almost 7000 female hormone pellet procedures and over 2100 male pellet procedures.

What I found in the data was over 80 percent of the females since 2012 remained on therapy for greater than five years, and 50 percent of those females remained on therapy for the entire 10-year span. The most common reason for stopping pellet therapy was either cost, relocation, or unfounded fears, usually from their primary healthcare provider. There were zero reported adverse events, such as deaths or hospitalizations in women or men; the reported incidences of invasive breast cancer were markedly reduced compared to the general population averages. The nuisance side effects that were reported were dose dependent, manageable, and did not prohibit, in most cases, continuation of the therapy. Nuisance side effects are typically hair growth in areas females do not want, facial breakouts, water retention, and abnormal uterine bleeding. Men rarely have side effects, but a typical side effect they might experience when they initiate therapy is temporary water retention, as testosterone stimulates muscle growth, and muscle growth causes water retention.

CHAPTER 12

FINAL THOUGHTS

I've just scratched the surface of the surface in this book of how vitally important paying attention to these life-giving molecules called hormones is. So many people, health care providers included, hear the word "hormone" and think of menstrual cycles, pregnancy, and menopause in females and sexual function in males. As you now understand, it is so much more than that!

I am confident you now grasp the impact sex hormones play not only in decreasing the common symptoms of hormone decline - depression, anxiety, irritability, mood swings, brain fog, trouble focusing, memory loss, insomnia, chronic pain, weight gain, decreased sex drive- but also in chronic disease prevention. Gut health and the effects of our diet on hormone production, metabolism, function, and excretion cannot be emphasized enough! A well-rounded hormone treatment plan will not only evaluate symptoms and blood levels but also gut health and nutrition status. I hope that you have also gotten some insights about other key hormones like thyroid, DHEA, and melatonin and how important all of these hormones are in working together to keep our bodies functioning optimally for a long time!

Some people, including healthcare providers, have asked me the question "Shouldn't I just age naturally?" I believe this was true in another time, when humans didn't live on such a toxic planet - from the air, water, and food to the news, social media, and internet- toxicity from chemicals, negative news and thoughts wreak havoc on our health and well-being. Outside negative stimuli inundate the mind, body, and soul.

Unless you live on an island - away from technology and industry; away from toxic news, thoughts, and people; eat foods grown in their natural environment, seasonally in rich soil without chemicals (including meat, fish, and poultry) and are physically active every day, growing old naturally and gracefully is essentially a myth. Don't get me wrong, we can certainly try and get as close to optimal heath as naturally as possible by nurturing our minds, bodies, and souls in all of the ways I have mentioned. However what I have found over the years of helping people address the root cause of common complaints- fatigue, lack of stamina, anxiety, depression, weight gain, chronic diseases, pain, etc.- is many people view becom-

"Unless you live on an island- away from technology and industry; away from toxic news, thoughts, and people; eat foods grown in their natural environment, seasonally in rich soil without chemicals (including meat, fish, and poultry) and are physically active every day, growing old naturally and gracefully is essentially a myth."

ing well as just too much work. In my experience, many people want change, *but they don't want to change.*

But I can tell you, much like many of the stories I have shared in this book, once you optimize your hormones not only clinically with natural hormone therapy, but also being mindful of hormone metabolism, excretion and eliminating endocrine disruptors, the journey of becoming well becomes less daunting and more necessary. Once you begin to feel good and function the way your body is designed, it's almost impossible to go backwards.

"Once you begin to feel good and function the way your body is designed, it's almost impossible to go backwards."

The name of my clinics and the network of trained practitioners is EVEXIAS, which is Greek for wellness. Miriam-Webster defines wellness as "the quality or state of being in good health especially as an *actively* sought goal." The Cambridge dictionary defines wellness as "the state of being healthy, especially when it is something that you *actively* try to achieve". And dictionary.com describes wellness as "the quality or state of being healthy in body and mind, especially as the result of *deliberate effort;* an approach to healthcare that emphasizes preventing illness and prolonging life, as opposed to emphasizing treating diseases". *Note each definition of wellness describes an intentionality on our part.*

Being well doesn't happen naturally, not in our current world anyway, it takes effort; it takes an action on the part of the

"Being well doesn't happen naturally, not in our current world anyway, it takes effort; it takes an action on the part of the individual."

individual. Each choice you make- from your food to your thoughts to your relationships - impacts your overall wellness. YOU are in the driver's seat; YOU get to choose the quality of your life.

FOOD FOR THOUGHT

Do you take time to nurture your body with positive ions that come from nature - waterfalls, oceans, streams, mountains, digging or planting in unspoiled dirt? Do you surround yourself with positive people who encourage you? Do you laugh every day? Do you take time away from electronics (phones, tablets, computers) and social media? Do you move your body every day in some way? Do you prepare and eat healthy, unprocessed homemade meals with family or community often? Do you sleep seven hours most nights with no light stimulus? Do you do something you love every day? Do you meditate, pray, have quiet time or some other connection to your higher power daily? *This is how God designed us to be and live.*

Hundreds of patients have crossed the threshold of my clinics in Texas, as well as those of the nationwide network of providers who have been trained in these therapies, near to tears with relief that someone finally listened to them and understands they aren't "normal," and there is some light at the end of the tunnel.

So many people across the country, and likely the globe, needlessly suffer from a lack of total body wellness that manifests as symptoms that have a root cause in many of the hormone deficiencies or other aspects of health I have discussed. Many have gone to several healthcare practitioners, and have tried a myriad of remedies, to no avail. It is my sincere prayer, if you are one of those people, that reading this book has given you some resources, but mostly hope that there is an answer and has prompted you to embark on your own journey of achieving optimal health and wellness.

REFERENCES BY CHAPTERS

INTRODUCTION & ESTROGEN

1. Borrás C, Mas-Bargues C, Román-Domínguez A, Sanz-Ros J, Gimeno-Mallench L, Inglés M, Gambini J, Viña J. BCL-xL, a Mitochondrial Protein Involved in Successful Aging: From *C. elegans* to Human Centenarians. Int J Mol Sci. 2020 Jan 9;21(2):418. doi: 10.3390/ijms21020418. PMID: 31936510; PMCID: PMC7014191.

2. Burnett-Bowie, S. A. M., McKay, E. A., Lee, H., & Leder, B. Z. (2009). Effects of aromatase inhibition on bone mineral density and bone turnover in older men with low testosterone levels. *The Journal of Clinical Endocrinology & Metabolism*, *94*(12), 4785-4792.

3. Carlson, M. C., Zandi, P. P., Plassman, B. L., Tschanz, J. T., Welsh-Bohmer, K. A., Steffens, D. C., ... & Breitner, J. C. S. (2001). Hormone replacement therapy and reduced cognitive decline in older women: the Cache County Study. *Neurology*, *57*(12), 2210-2216.

4. Cerri, S., Mus, L., & Blandini, F. (2019). Parkinson's disease in women and men: what's the difference?. *Journal of Parkinson's disease*, *9*(3), 501-515.

5. Chlebowski, R. T., Anderson, G. L., Aragaki, A. K., Manson, J. E., Stefanick, M. L., Pan, K., ... & Prentice, R. L. (2020). Association of menopausal hormone therapy with breast cancer incidence and mortality during long-term follow-up of the women's health initiative randomized clinical trials. *Jama, 324*(4), 369-380.

6. Davis, S. R., Walker, K. Z., & Strauss, B. J. (2000). Effects of estradiol with and without testosterone on body composition and relationships with lipids in postmenopausal women. *Menopause, 7*(6), 395-401.

7. Decker DA, Pettinga JE, VanderVelde
N, et al. Estrogen replacement therapy in breast cancer survivors: a matched-controlled series. Menopause. 2003 Jul-Aug;10(4):277-85.

8. de Lignieres B, de Vathaire
F, Fournier S, et al. Combined hormone replacement therapy and risk of breast cancer in a French cohort study of 3175 women. Climacteric. 2002;5:332-340.

9. DeNeui, T., Berg, J., & Howson, A. (2019). Best practices in care for menopausal patients: 16 years after the Women's Health Initiative. *Journal of the American Association of Nurse Practitioners, 31*(7), 420-427.

10. Dubal, D. B., & Wise, P. M. (2022). Estrogen and neuroprotection: from clinical observations to molecular mechanisms. *Dialogues in clinical neuroscience.*

11. E. Farish et al Acta Endocinoligca 1984, 106: 116-120 The Effects of Hormone Implants on Serum Lipoproteins and Steroid Hormones in Bilaterally Oophorectomized Women.

12. Fleta-Asín, B. (2007). Estrogens and cardiovascular disease in the male. *Revista espanola de cardiologia, 60*(06), 667-668.

13. Greendale, G. A., Espeland, M., Slone, S., Marcus, R., & Barrett-Connor, E. (2002). Bone mass response to discontinuation of long-term hormone replacement therapy: results from the Postmenopausal

Estrogen/Progestin Interventions (PEPI) Safety Follow-up Study. *Archives of internal medicine*, *162*(6), 665-672.

14. Hodis, H. N., Mack, W. J., Shoupe, D., Azen, S. P., Stanczyk, F. Z., Hwang-Levine, J., ... & Henderson, V. W. (2014). Testing the menopausal hormone therapy timing hypothesis: the Early versus Late Intervention Trial with Estradiol.

15. Henderson, V. W. (2014). Alzheimer's disease: review of hormone therapy trials and implications for treatment and prevention after menopause. The Journal of steroid biochemistry and molecular biology, 142, 99-106.

16. Hampel, H., Hardy, J., Blennow, K., Chen, C., Perry, G., Kim, S. H., ... & Vergallo, A. (2021). The amyloid-β pathway in Alzheimer's disease. *Molecular psychiatry,* 26(10), 5481-5503.

17. Jancin B. HRT Safe for Survivors of Early-Stage Breast Ca. Family Practice News. 2001 Jun 1.

18. Jett, S., Schelbaum, E., Jang, G., Boneu Yepez, C., Dyke, J. P., Pahlajani, S., ... & Mosconi, L. (2022). Ovarian steroid hormones: A long overlooked but critical contributor to brain aging and Alzheimer's disease. *Frontiers in Aging Neuroscience*, 14, 948219.

19. Jett, S., Malviya, N., Schelbaum, E., Jang, G., Jahan, E., Clancy, K., ... & Mosconi, L. (2022). Endogenous and exogenous estrogen exposures: how women's reproductive health can drive brain aging and inform Alzheimer's prevention. *Frontiers in Aging Neuroscience*, 150.

20. K. A., Mayer, L. S., Steffens, D. C., ... & Cache County Memory Study Investigators. (2002). Hormone replacement therapy and incidence of Alzheimer disease in older women: the Cache County Study. *Jama*, *288*(17), 2123-2129.

21. Lee, Y. H., Cha, J., Chung, S. J., Yoo, H. S., Sohn, Y. H., Ye, B. S., & Lee, P. H. (2019). Beneficial effect of estrogen on nigrostriatal dopaminergic neurons in drug-naïve postmenopausal Parkinson's disease. *Scientific reports*, *9*(1), 1-9.

22. Lephart, E. D., & Naftolin, F. (2021). Menopause and the skin: Old favorites and new innovations in cosmeceuticals for estrogen-deficient skin. *Dermatology and Therapy*, *11*, 53-69.

23. Levgur M. Hormone therapy for women after breast cancer. J of Reprod Med. 2004 Jul;49(7):510-26.

24. Lobo, R. A., Pickar, J. H., Stevenson, J. C., Mack, W. J., & Hodis, H. N. (2016). Back to the future: hormone replacement therapy as part of a prevention strategy for women at the onset of menopause. *Atherosclerosis*, *254*, 282-290.

25. Luine, V. N. (2014). Estradiol and cognitive function: past, present and future. Hormones and behavior, 66(4), 602-618.

26. Peters GN, Fodera T, Sabol J, et al. Estrogen replacement therapy after breast cancer: a 12-year follow-up. Ann Surg Oncol. 2001 Dec;8(10):828-32.

27. Petrone, A. Wise, P. M., Suzuki, S., & Brown, C. M. (2023). Estradiol: a hormone with diverse and contradictory neuroprotective actions. *Dialogues in clinical neuroscience.*

28. Pike, C. J. (1999). Estrogen Modulates Neuronal Bcl-xl Expression and β-Amyloid-Induced Apoptosis: Relevance to Alzheimer's Disease. Journal of neurochemistry, 72(4), 1552-1563.

29. Mahmoodzadeh, S., Leber, J., Zhang, X., Jaisser, F., Messaoudi, S., Morano, I., ... & Regitz-Zagrosek, V. (2014). Cardiomyocyte-specific estrogen receptor alpha increases angiogenesis, lymphangiogenesis and reduces fibrosis in the female mouse heart post-myocardial infarction. *Journal of cell science & therapy*, *5*(1), 153.

30. Maioli, S., Leander, K., Nilsson, P., & Nalvarte, I. (2021). Estrogen receptors and the aging brain. *Essays in Biochemistry*, *65*(6), 913-925.

31. Menazza, S., & Murphy, E. (2016). The expanding complexity of estrogen receptor signaling in the cardiovascular system. *Circulation research*, *118*(6), 994-1007.

32. Mikkola, T. S., Savolainen-Peltonen, H., Venetkoski, M., & Ylikorkala, O. (2017). New evidence for cardiac benefit of postmenopausal hormone therapy. *Climacteric*, *20*(1), 5-10.

33. Mikkola, T. S., Savolainen-Peltonen, H., Tuomikoski, P., Hoti, F., Vattulainen, P., Gissler, M., & Ylikorkala, O. (2016). Lower death risk for vascular dementia than for Alzheimer's disease with postmenopausal hormone therapy users. The Journal of Clinical Endocrinology & Metabolism, 102(3), 870-877.

34. Natrajan PK, Gambrell RD. Estrogen replacement therapy in patients with early breast cancer. Am J Obstet Gynecol. 2002 Aug;187(2):289-94.

35. Natrajan PK, Soumakis K, Gambrell RD Jr. Estrogen replacement therapy in women with previous breast cancer. Am J Obstet Gynecol. 1999 Aug;181(2):288-95.

36. Notelovitz, M., Johnston, M, Smith, S, & Kitchens, C. (1987). Metabolic and hormonal effects of 25 mg and 50 mg 17b-estradiol implants in surgically menopausal women. *Obstet Gynecol*, *70*, 749-54.

37. Rzepecki, A. K., Murase, J. E., Juran, R., Fabi, S. G., & McLellan, B. N. (2019). Estrogen-deficient skin: the role of topical therapy. *International journal of women's dermatology*, *5*(2), 85-90.

38. Sarrel, P. M., Njike, V. Y., Vinante, V., & Katz, D. L. (2013). The mortality toll of estrogen avoidance: an analysis of excess deaths among hysterectomized women aged 50 to 59 years. American journal of public health, 103(9), 1583-1588.

39. Savvas, M., Studd, J. W. W., Norman, S., Leather, A. T., Garnett, T. J., & Fogelman, I. (1992). Increase in bone mass after one year of percutaneous oestradiol and testosterone implants in post-menopausal women who have previously received long-term oral oestrogens. BJOG: *An International Journal of Obstetrics & Gynaecology*, 99(9), 757-760.

40. Shao, H., Breitner, J. C., Whitmer, R. A., Wang, J., Hayden, K., Wengreen, H., ... & Welsh-Bohmer, K. (2012). Hormone therapy and

Alzheimer disease dementia New findings from the Cache County Study. *Neurology*, *79*(18), 1846-1852.

41. Simpkins, J. W., & Barr, T. L. (2014). 17β-estradiol and inflammation: implications for ischemic stroke. Aging and disease, 5(5), 340.

42. Song, Y. J., Li, S. R., Li, X. W., Chen, X., Wei, Z. X., Liu, Q. S., & Cheng, Y. (2020). The effect of estrogen replacement therapy on Alzheimer's disease and Parkinson's disease in postmenopausal women: a meta-analysis. *Frontiers in Neuroscience*, *14*, 157.

43. Thadathil, N., Xiao, J., Hori, R., Alway, S. E., & Khan, M. M. (2021). Brain selective estrogen treatment protects dopaminergic neurons and preserves behavioral function in MPTP-induced mouse model of Parkinson's disease. *Journal of Neuroimmune Pharmacology*, *16*, 667-678.

44. Thornton, M. J. (2013). Estrogens and aging skin. *Dermato-endocrinology*, *5*(2), 264-270.

45. Tuomikoski, P., Salomaa, V., Havulinna, A., Airaksinen, J., Ketonen, M., Koukkunen, H., ... & Mikkola, T. S. (2016). Decreased mortality risk due to first acute coronary syndrome in women with postmenopausal hormone therapy use. *Maturitas*, *94*, 106-109.

46. US health ranking https://www.apha.org/topics-and-issues/health-rankings

47. Wilkinson, H. N., & Hardman, M. J. (2017). The role of estrogen in cutaneous ageing and repair. *Maturitas*, *103*, 60-64.

48. Wilkinson, H. N., & Hardman, M. J. (2021). A role for estrogen in skin ageing and dermal biomechanics. *Mechanisms of Ageing and Development*, *197*, 111513.

49. Wu, S., & Weng, X. (1992). Therapeutic effect of andriol on serum lipids and apolipoproteins in elderly male coronary heart disease patients. Chinese medical sciences journal= Chung-kuo i hsueh k'o hsueh tsa chih, 7(3), 137-141.

50. Wu, M., Li, M., Yuan, J., Liang, S., Chen, Z., Ye, M., ... & Bhagavathula, A. S. (2020). Postmenopausal hormone therapy and Alzheimer's disease, dementia, and Parkinson's disease: A systematic review and time-response meta-analysis. *Pharmacological research*, *155*, 104693.

51. Yoon, B. K., Chin, J., Kim, J. W., Shin, M. H., Ahn, S., Lee, D. Y., ... & Na, D. L. (2018). Menopausal hormone therapy and mild cognitive impairment: a randomized, placebo-controlled trial. Menopause, 25(8), 870-876.

52. Zandi, P. P., Carlson, M. C., Plassman, B. L., Welsh-Bohmer, K. A., Mayer, L. S., Steffens, D. C., ... & Cache County Memory Study Investigators. (2002). Hormone replacement therapy and incidence of Alzheimer disease in older women: the Cache County Study. *Jama*, *288*(17), 2123-2129.

53. Zhu, Y., Zhang, Q., Zhang, W., Li, N., Dai, Y., Tu, J., ... & Wang, R. (2017). Protective effect of 17β-estradiol upon hippocampal spine density and cognitive function in an animal model of vascular dementia. *Scientific reports*, 7, 42660.

PROGESTERONE

1. Berent-Spillson, A., Briceno, E., Pinsky, A., Simmen, A., Persad, C. C., Zubieta, J. K., & Smith, Y. R. (2015). Distinct cognitive effects of estrogen and progesterone in menopausal women. Psychoneuroendocrinology, 59, 25-36.

2. Campagnoli C, Abba C, Amgroggio S, Peris C. Pregnancy, progesterone and progestins in relation to breast cancer risk. J of Steroid Biochem& Molecular Biol. 2005;97:441-450.

3. DeNeui, T., Berg, J., & Howson, A. (2019). Best practices in care for menopausal patients: 16 years after the Women's Health Initiative. *Journal of the American Association of Nurse Practitioners*, *31*(7), 420-427.

4. Foidart JM, Colin C, Denoo
X, et al. Estradiol and progesterone regulate the proliferation of human breast epithelial cells. Fertil Steril. 1998 May;69(5):963-9.

5. Fournier A, Berrino F, Riboli
E, et al. Breast cancer risk in relation to different types of hormone replacement therapy in the E3N-EPIC cohort. Int J Cancer. 2005 Apr 10;114(3):448-54.

6. Ghandehari, S., Matusov, Y., Pepkowitz, S., Stein, D., Kaderi, T., Narayanan, D., ... & Lewis, M. (2021). Progesterone in addition to standard of care vs standard of care alone in the treatment of men hospitalized with moderate to severe COVID-19: a randomized, controlled pilot trial. *Chest*, *160*(1), 74-84.

7. Gizard F, Robillard R, Gervois
P, et al. Progesterone inhibits human breast cancer cell growth through transcriptional upregulation of the cyclin-dependent kinase inhibitor p27Kip1 gene. FEBS Lett. 2005 Oct 24;579(25):5535-41.

8. Nagy, B., Szekeres-Barthó, J., Kovács, G. L., Sulyok, E., Farkas, B., Várnagy, Á., ... & Bódis, J. (2021). Key to life: physiological role and clinical implications of progesterone. *International Journal of Molecular Sciences*, *22*(20), 11039.

9. Oettel, M., & Mukhopadhyay, A. K. (2004). Progesterone: the forgotten hormone in men?. *The Aging Male*, *7*(3), 236-257.

10. Prior, J. C. (2018). Progesterone for treatment of symptomatic menopausal women. Climacteric, 21(4), 358-365.

11. Sitruk-Ware, R. (2018). Non-clinical studies of progesterone. Climacteric, 21(4), 315-320

12. Wood CE, Register TC, Lees CJ, et al. Effects of estradiol with micronized progesterone or medroxyprogesterone acetate on risk markers for breast cancer in postmenopausal monkeys. Breast Cancer Res Treat. 2007 Jan;101(2):125-34.

TESTOSTERONE

1. Alberts B, Johnson A, Lewis J, et al. Molecular Biology of the Cell. 4th edition. New York: Garland Science; 2002. Blood Vessels and Endothelial Cells. Available from: https://www.ncbi.nlm.nih.gov/books/NBK26848/

2. Al-Azzawi, F., Bitzer, J., Brandenburg, U., Castelo-Branco, C., Graziottin, A., Kenemans, P., ... & Zahradnik, H. P. (2010). Therapeutic options for postmenopausal female sexual dysfunction. *Climacteric*, *13*(2), 103-120.

3. Baldassarre, M., Perrone, A. M., Giannone, F. A., Armillotta, F., Battaglia, C., Costantino, A., ... & Meriggiola, M. C. (2013). Androgen receptor expression in the human vagina under different physiological and treatment conditions. *International journal of impotence research*, *25*(1), 7-11.

4. Basson, R. (2010). Testosterone therapy for reduced libido in women. *Therapeutic advances in endocrinology and metabolism*, *1*(4), 155-164.

5. Boni C, Pagano M, Panebianco M et al. Therapeutic Activity of Testosterone in Metastatic Breast Cancer. Anticancer research. 2014;34:1287-1290.

6. Burger HG. Androgen production in women. Fertility and sterility. 2002;77:3-5.

7. Chen, X., Zhang, J., & Wang, X. (2016). Hormones in pain modulation and their clinical implications for pain control: a critical review. Hormones, 15(3), 313-320.

8. Chistiakov, D. A., Myasoedova, V. A., Melnichenko, A. A., Grechko, A. V., & Orekhov, A. N. (2018). Role of androgens in cardiovascular pathology. *Vascular health and risk management*, *14*, 283.

9. Ciocca, G., Limoncin, E., Carosa, E., Di Sante, S., Gravina, G. L., Mollaioli, D., ... & Jannini, E. A. (2016). Is testosterone a food for the brain?. *Sexual*

10. Daka, B., Langer, R. D., Larsson, C. A., Rosén, T., Jansson, P. A., Råstam, L., & Lindblad, U. (2015). Low concentrations of serum testosterone predict acute myocardial infarction in men with type 2 diabetes mellitus. *BMC endocrine disorders*, *15*(1), 35 .

11. Davis, S. R., & Tran, J. (2001). Testosterone influences libido and well being in women. *Trends in Endocrinology & Metabolism*, *12*(1), 33-37.

12. Debing, E., Peeters, E., Duquet, W., Poppe, K., Velkeniers, B., & Van den Brande, P. (2007). Endogenous sex hormone levels in postmenopausal women undergoing carotid artery endarterectomy. European journal of endocrinology, 156(6), 687-693.

13. DeNeui, T., Gilder, R., & Michael, J. (2018). *Compliance with Post-Intervention Follow-up in the Depressive Pre, Peri and Post-Menopausal Client: A QI Initiative*. Unpublished Capstone Project, University of Texas at Arlington

14. Dimitrakakis, C., & Bondy, C. (2009). Androgens and the breast. Breast cancer research, 11(5), 212.

15. Donovitz, G., & Cotten, M. (2021). Breast Cancer Incidence Reduction in Women Treated with Subcutaneous Testosterone: Testosterone Therapy and Breast Cancer Incidence Study. *European journal of breast health*, *17*(2), 150

16. Ebinger, M., Sievers, C., Ivan, D., Schneider, H. J., & Stalla, G. K. (2008). Is there a neuroendocrinological rationale for testosterone as a therapeutic option in depression? *Journal of Psychopharmacology*. *23*(7), 841-853.

17. Feldhaus-Dahir, M. (2009). Testosterone for the treatment of hypoactive sexual desire disorder: part II. *Urologic nursing*, *29*(5), 3869.

18. Fountas, A., Chai, S. T., Kourkouti, C., & Karavitaki, N. (2018). Mechanisms of endocrinology: Endocrinology of opioids. *European journal of endocrinology*, *179*(4), R183-R196.

19. Glaser, R., & Dimitrakakis, C. (2015). Testosterone and breast cancer prevention. Maturitas, 82(3), 291-295.

20. Glaser, R. L., & Dimitrakakis, C. (2014). Rapid response of breast cancer to neoadjuvant intramammary testosterone-anastrozole therapy: neoadjuvant hormone therapy in breast cancer. Menopause (New York, NY), 21(6), 673.

21. Glaser, R. L., & Dimitrakakis, C. (2014). Rapid response of breast cancer to neoadjuvant intramammary testosterone-anastrozole therapy: neoadjuvant hormone therapy in breast cancer. Menopause (New York, NY), 21(6), 673.

22. Glaser, R., & Dimitrakakis, C. (2015). Testosterone and breast cancer prevention. Maturitas, 82(3), 291-295.

23. Glaser, R. L., & Dimitrakakis, C. (2013). Reduced breast cancer incidence in women treated with subcutaneous testosterone, or testosterone with anastrozole: a prospective, observational study. Maturitas, 76(4), 342-349.

24. Glaser, Rebecca & York, Anne & Dimitrakakis, Constantine. (2019). Incidence of invasive breast cancer in women treated with testosterone implants: a prospective 10-year cohort study. BMC Cancer. 19. 10.1186/s12885-019-6457-8.

25. Goldenberg, I.S. (1964). Testosterone Proionate Therapy in Breast Cancer. JAMA, 188(12). 117-120.

26. Goldstat, R., Briganti, E., Tran, J., Wolfe, R., & Davis, S. R. (2003). Transdermal testosterone therapy improves well-being, mood, and sexual function in premenopausal women. *Menopause*, *10*(5), 390-398.

27. Gururani, K., Jose, J., & George, P. V. (2016). Testosterone as a marker of coronary artery disease severity in middle aged males. *Indian heart journal*, *68*, S16-S20 .

28. Jovanovic, H., Kocoska-Maras, L., Rådestad, A. F., Halldin, C., Borg, J., Hirschberg, A. L., & Nordström, A. L. (2015). Effects of estrogen and testosterone treatment on serotonin transporter binding in the brain of surgically postmenopausal women–a PET study. *Neuroimage*, *106*, 47-54.

29. Kautz, H.D. & DeNosaquo, N. (1960). Report to the Council: Androgens and estrogens in the treatment of disseminated mammary carcinoma. JAMA, 172(12), 135-172.

30. Kay-Tee, K., & Chir, M. B. B. (2007). Endogenous testosterone and mortality due to all causes, cardiovascular disease, and cancer in men. Am Heart Association, 116, 2694-701.

31. Khaw, K. T., Dowsett, M., Folkerd, E., Bingham, S., Wareham, N., Luben, R., ... & Day, N. (2007). Endogenous testosterone and mortality due to all causes, cardiovascular disease, and cancer in men: European prospective investigation into cancer in Norfolk (EPIC-Norfolk) Prospective Population Study. Circulation, 116(23), 2694-2701.

32. Kimura NORIKO, Mizokami ATSUSHI, Oonuma TETSUTAROU, Sasano HIRONOBU, Nagura HIROSHI. Immunocytochemical localization of androgen receptor with polyclonal antibody in paraffin-embedded human tissues. Journal of Histochemistry & Cytochemistry. 1993;41:671-678.

33. Krapf, J. M., & Simon, J. A. (2009). The role of testosterone in the management of hypoactive sexual desire disorder in postmenopausal women. *Maturitas*, *63*(3), 213-219.

34. Kumsar, Ş., Kumsar, N. A., Sağlam, H. S., Köse, O., Budak, S., & Adsan, Ö. (2014). Testosterone levels and sexual function disorders in depressive female patients: effects of antidepressant treatment. *The journal of sexual medicine*, *11*(2), 529.

35. Labrie F. All sex steroids are made intracellularly in peripheral tissues by the mechanisms of intracrinology after menopause. The Journal of steroid biochemistry and molecular biology. 2015;145:133-138.

36. Labrie, F., Martel, C., & Pelletier, G. (2017). Is vulvovaginal atrophy due to a lack of both estrogens and androgens? *Menopause*, *24*(4), 452-461.

37. Lucas-Herald, A. K., Alves-Lopes, R., Montezano, A. C., Ahmed, S. F., & Touyz, R. M. (2017). Genomic and non-genomic effects of

androgens in the cardiovascular system: clinical implications. *Clinical Science, 131*(13), 1405-1418.

38. Longscope C. Adrenal and gonadal androgen secretion in normal female. J Clin Endocrinol Metab. 1986;15:213-228.

39. Malkin, C. J., Pugh, P. J., Morris, P. D., Kerry, K. E., Jones, R. D., Jones, T. H., & Channer, K. S. (2004). Testosterone replacement in hypogonadal men with angina improves ischemic threshold and quality of life. Heart, 90(8), 871-876.

40. Moretti, C., Lanzolla, G., Moretti, M., Gnessi, L., & Carmina, E. (2017). Androgens and hypertension in men and women: a unifying view. *Current hypertension reports, 19*(5), 44.

41. Malkin, C. J., Pugh, P. J., Morris, P. D., Kerry, K. E., Jones, R. D., Jones, T. H., & Channer, K. S. (2004). Testosterone replacement in hypogonadal men with angina improves ischemic threshold and quality of life. Heart, 90(8), 871-876.

42. Meaini L, Zucchi A World J Urol 2011 Nov 9 Urology 2006;68: 1263-67 International Journal of Impotence Research 2009;21;9-23 Ararwal et. al. J. Urology 2005.

43. Morgentaler, A. (2012). Goodbye androgen hypothesis, hello saturation model. *European urology, 62*(5), 765-767.2005

44. Morgentaler, A., Lipshultz, L. I., Bennett, R., Sweeney, M., Avila, D., & Khera, M. (2011). Testosterone therapy in men with untreated prostate cancer. The Journal of urology, 185(4), 1256-1261.

45. Nappi, R. E., Detaddei, S., Ferdeghini, F., Brundu, B., Sommacal, A., & Polatti, F. (2003). Role of testosterone in feminine sexuality. *Journal of Endocrinological Investigation, 26*(3 Suppl), 97-101.

46. Nappi, R. E. (2015). Why are there no FDA-approved treatments for female sexual dysfunction?

47. Natrajan, P. K., Soumakis, K., & Gambrell Jr, R. D. (1999). Estrogen replacement therapy in women with previous breast cancer. *American journal of obstetrics and gynecology, 181*(2), 288-295.

48. Notelovitz, M., Johnston, M, Smith, S, & Kitchens, C. (1987). Metabolic and hormonal effects of 25 mg and 50 mg 17b-estradiol implants in surgically menopausal women. Obstet Gynecol, 70, 749-54.

49. Pastuszak, A. W., Pearlman, A. M., Lai, W. S., Godoy, G., Sathyamoorthy, K., Liu, J. S., ... & Khera, M. (2013). Testosterone replacement therapy in patients with prostate cancer after radical prostatectomy. The Journal of urology, 190(2), 639-644.

50. Palacios, S. (2007). Androgens and female sexual function. *Maturitas*, *57*(1), 61-65.

51. Pastuszak, A. W., Pearlman, A. M., Lai, W. S., Godoy, G., Sathyamoorthy, K., Liu, J. S., ... & Khera, M. (2013). Testosterone replacement therapy in patients with prostate cancer after radical prostatectomy. The Journal of urology, 190(2), 639-644.

52. Pluchino, N., Carmignani, A., Cubeddu, A., Santoro, A., Cela, V., & Alcala, T. E. (2013). Androgen therapy in women: for whom and when. *Archives of gynecology and obstetrics*, *288*(4), 731-737.

53. Quigley CA, Bellis AD, Marschke KB, El-Awady MK, Wilson EM, French FS. Androgen Receptor Defects: Historical, Clinical, and Molecular Perspectives*. Endocrine reviews. 1995;16:271-321.

54. Richards M. Hidden in Plain Sight: A Real Solution to the Diseases of Aging and the Imploding Medicare System.

55. Said Ghandour, Rhonda Voskuhl & Michael Schumacher (2014) The androgen receptor as a therapeutic target for myelin repair in demyelinating diseases, Expert Review of Endocrinology & Metabolism, 9:1, 5-7, DOI: 10.1586/17446651.2014.861740

56. Savvas, M., Studd, J. W. W., Norman, S., Leather, A. T., Garnett, T. J., & Fogelman, I. (1992). Increase in bone mass after one year of percutaneous oestradiol and testosterone implants in post-menopausal women who have previously received long-term oral oestrogens. BJOG: An International Journal of Obstetrics & Gynaecology.

57. Scavello, I., Maseroli, E., Di Stasi, V., & Vignozzi, L. (2019). Sexual health in menopause. *Medicina, 55*(9), 559.

58. Schwenkhagen, A., & Studd, J. (2009). Role of testosterone in the treatment of hypoactive sexual desire disorder. *Maturitas, 63*(2), 152-159.

59. Seidman, S. N., & Roose, S. P. (2006). The sexual effects of testosterone replacement in depressed men: randomized, placebo-controlled clinical trial. *Journal of sex & marital therapy, 32*(3), 267-273.

60. Simon, D., Charles, M. A., Nahoul, K., Orssaud, G., Kremski, J., Hully, V., ... & Eschwege, E. (1997). Association between plasma total testosterone and cardiovascular risk factors in healthy adult men: The Telecom Study. The Journal of Clinical Endocrinology & Metabolism, 82(2), 682-685.

61. Studd, J., & Panay, N. (2004). Hormones and depression in women. *Climacteric, 7*(4), 338-346.

62. Studd, J., Savvas, M., Waston, N., Garnett, T., Fogelman, I., & Cooper, D. (1990). The relationship between plasma estradiol and the increase in bone density in postmenopausal women after treatment with subcutaneous hormone implants. American journal of obstetrics and gynecology, 163(5), 1474-1479.

63. Takeda, H., Chodak, G., Mutchnik, S., Nakamoto, T., & Chang, C. (1990). Immunohistochemical localization of androgen receptors with mono-and polyclonal antibodies to androgen receptor. *Journal of Endocrinology, 126*(1), 17-NP.

64. Tennant, F., & Lichota, L. (2010). Testosterone replacement in chronic pain patients. *Pract. Pain Manage, 10*(6), 12-15.

65. Traish, A. M., Vignozzi, L., Simon, J. A., Goldstein, I., & Kim, N. N. (2018). Role of androgens in female genitourinary tissue structure and function: implications in the genitourinary syndrome of menopause. *Sexual Medicine Reviews, 6*(4), 558-571.

66. Traish, A. M., Kim, N., Min, K., Munarriz, R., & Goldstein, I. (2002). Role of androgens in female genital sexual arousal: receptor expression, structure, and function. *Fertility and sterility*, *77*, 11-18.

67. Uloko, M., Rahman, F., Puri, L. I., & Rubin, R. S. (2022). The clinical management of testosterone replacement therapy in postmenopausal women with hypoactive sexual desire disorder: a review. *International Journal of Impotence Research*, *34*(7), 635-641.

68. Vest, R. S., & Pike, C. J. (2013). Gender, sex steroid hormones, and Alzheimer's disease. *Hormones and behavior*, *63*(2), 301-307.

69. White, K. C. (2017). Transdermal Testosterone For Menopause-Related Hyposexual Desire Disorder: Current Guidelines And Provider Perceptions, Knowledge, And Practice.

70. Wilson CM, McPhaul MJ. A and B forms of the androgen receptor are expressed in a variety of human tissues. Molecular and cellular endocrinology. 1996;120:51-57.

71. Zarrouf, F. A., Artz, S., Griffith, J., Sirbu, C., & Kommor, M. (2009). Testosterone and depression: systematic review and meta-analysis. *Journal of Psychiatric Practice®*, *15*(4), 289-305.

THYROID

1. Appetecchia, M. (2005). Effects on bone mineral density by treatment of benign nodular goiter with mildly suppressive doses of L-thyroxine in a cohort women study. Hormone Research in Paediatrics, 64(6), 293-298.

2. Azizi, F., Amouzegar, A., Mehran, L., & Abdi, H. (2020). LT4 and slow release T3 combination: optimum therapy for hypothyroidism?. *International journal of endocrinology and metabolism*, *18*(2).

3. Baldini, M., Gallazzi, M., Orsatti, A., Fossati, S., Leonardi, P., & Cantalamessa, L. (2002). Treatment of benign nodular goitre with mildly suppressive doses of L-thyroxine: effects on bone mineral density and on nodule size. Journal of internal medicine, 251(5), 407-414.

4. Bertani, L., Tricò, D., Pugliese, D., Privitera, G., Linsalata, G., Zanzi, F., ... & Costa, F. (2021). Serum triiodothyronine-to-thyroxine (T3/T4) ratio predicts therapeutic outcome to biological therapies in elderly IBD patients. *Alimentary Pharmacology & Therapeutics,* 53(2), 273-280.

5. Büber, İ., Eraydın, A., Sevgican, C. İ., Tekin, I., Kılıç, İ. D., & Fenkçi, S. M. (2023). The Effects of Combination Treatment T4 and T3 on Diastolic Functions and Atrial Conduction Time in Women with Low T3: A short term Follow-up Study.

6. Carbery, I., Lin, S., Chanchlani, N., Janjua, M., Nice, R., McDonald, T. J., ... & Selinger, C. P. (2023). P649 Does serum triiodothyronine-to-thyroxine (T3/T4) ratio predict therapeutic outcome to anti-TNF therapies in biologic-naïve patients with active luminal Crohn's disease?. *Journal of Crohn's and Colitis, 17*(Supplement_1), i778-i778.

7. Cerillo, A. G., Storti, S., Kallushi, E., Haxhiademi, D., Miceli, A., Murzi, M., ... & Iervasi, G. (2014). The low triiodothyronine syndrome: a strong predictor of low cardiac output and death in patients undergoing coronary artery bypass grafting. The Annals of thoracic surgery, 97(6), 2089-2095.

8. Desai, A., Rothberger, G., Valestra, P. K., Khalilah, D., Calixte, R., & Shapiro, L. (2018). Low Free T3 Is Associated with Worse Outcomes in Patients with Acute Respiratory Failure Requiring Invasive Mechanical Ventilation. In A24. CRITICAL CARE: ARDS AND ACUTE RESPIRATORY FAILURE-CAN WE DO BETTER? (pp. A1134-A1134). American Thoracic Society.

9. Escobar-Morreale, H. F., Del Rey, F. E., Obregón, M. J., & de Escobar, G. M. (1996). Only the combined treatment with

thyroxine and triiodothyronine ensures euthyroidism in all tissues of the thyroidectomized rat. *Endocrinology*, *137*(6), 2490-2502.

10. Escobar-Morreale, H. F., Botella-Carretero, J. I., del Rey, F. E., & de Escobar, G. M. (2005). Treatment of hypothyroidism with combinations of levothyroxine plus liothyronine. The Journal of Clinical Endocrinology & Metabolism, 90(8), 4946-4954.

11. Ettleson, M. D., & Bianco, A. C. (2020). Individualized Therapy for Hypothyroidism: Is T4 Enough for Everyone?. *J Clin Endocrinol Metab*, *105*(9), 1-15.

12. Fraser, W. D., Biggart, E. M., O'Reilly, D. S., Gray, H. W., McKillop, J. H., & Thomson, J. A. (1986). Are biochemical tests of thyroid function of any value in monitoring patients receiving thyroxine replacement?. *Br Med J (Clin Res Ed)*, *293*(6550), 808-810.

13. Friedberg, R. C., Souers, R., Wagar, E. A., Stankovic, A. K., & Valenstein, P. N. (2007). The origin of reference intervals: a College of American Pathologists Q-Probes study of "normal ranges" used in 163 clinical laboratories. *Archives of pathology & laboratory medicine*, *131*(3), 348-357.

14. Gereben, B., Zeöld, A., Dentice, M., Salvatore, D., & Bianco, A. C. (2008). Activation and inactivation of thyroid hormone by deiodinases: local action with general consequences. Cellular and Molecular Life Sciences, 65(4), 570-590.

15. Huang, X., Zhang, H., Qu, C., Liu, Y., Bian, C., & Xu, Y. (2019). Depression and insomnia are closely associated with thyroid hormone levels in chronic hepatitis B. Medical Science Monitor: International Medical Journal of Experimental and Clinical Research, 25, 2672.

16. Ichiki, T. (2016). Thyroid hormone and vascular remodeling. *Journal of atherosclerosis and thrombosis*, *23*(3), 266-275.

17. Ihnatowicz, P., Drywień, M., Wątor, P., & Wojsiat, J. (2020). The importance of nutritional factors and dietary management of

Hashimoto's thyroiditis. *Annals of agricultural and environmental medicine*, *27*(2), 184-193.

18. Jonklaas, J. (2017). Persistent hypothyroid symptoms in a patient with a normal thyroid stimulating hormone level. Current opinion in endocrinology, diabetes, and obesity, 24(5), 356.

19. Kahaly, G. J. (2023). Therapeutic Use of Levothyroxine: A Historical Perspective. 70 Years of Levothyroxine, 1-11.

20. Kelly, T. F., & Lieberman, D. Z. (2009). Long term augmentation with T3 in refractory major depression. Journal of affective disorders, 115(1-2), 230-233.

21. Lang, X., Li, Y., Zhang, D., Zhang, Y., Wu, N., & Zhang, Y. (2022). FT3/FT4 ratio is correlated with all-cause mortality, cardiovascular mortality, and cardiovascular disease risk: NHANES 2007-2012. *Frontiers in Endocrinology*, *13*, 964822

22. Larsen,P. R., Bleich, H. L., & Moore, M. J. (1982). Thyroid-pituitary interaction: Feedback regulation of thyrotropin secretion by thyroid hormones. New Engl. J. Med.;(United States), 306(1).

23. Neves, J. S., Dias, C. V., Leitao, L., Vieira, M. B., Magrico, R., Oliveira, A. I., ... & Leite-Moreira, A. (2018, May). Low free T3 levels within the reference range independently predict cardiovascular mortality in the general population. In 20th European Congress of Endocrinology (Vol. 56). BioScientifica.

24. Pappa, T., & Refetoff, S. (2021). Resistance to thyroid hormone beta: a focused review. *Frontiers in endocrinology*, *12*, 656551.

25. Peterson, S. J., Cappola, A. R., Castro, M. R., Dayan, C. M., Farwell, A. P., Hennessey, J. V., ... & Taylor, P. N. (2018). An online survey of hypothyroid patients demonstrates prominent dissatisfaction. Thyroid, 28(6), 707-721.

26. Pingitore, A., & Iervasi, G. (2005). Thyroid (dys) function in heart failure: is it a potential target for medical treatment?. Vascular health and risk management, 1(2),

27. Quan, M. L., Pasieka, J. L., & Rorstad, O. (2002). Bone mineral density in well-differentiated thyroid cancer patients treated with suppressive thyroxine: a systematic overview of the literature. Journal of surgical oncology, 79(1), 62-70.

28. Quinlan, P., Horvath, A., Wallin, A., & Svensson, J. (2019). Low serum concentration of free triiodothyronine (FT3) is associated with increased risk of Alzheimer's disease. *Psychoneuroendocrinology*, *99*, 112-119.

29. Reverter, J. L., Holgado, S., Alonso, N., Salinas, I., Granada, M. L., & Sanmarti, A. (2005). Lack of deleterious effect on bone mineral density of long-term thyroxine suppressive therapy for differentiated thyroid carcinoma. Endocrine-related cancer, 12(4), 973-981.

30. Strich, D., Karavani, G., Edri, S., & Gillis, D. (2016). TSH enhancement of FT4 to FT3 conversion is age dependent. *Eur J Endocrinol*, *175*(1), 49-54.

31. Tariq, A., Wert, Y., Cheriyath, P., & Joshi, R. (2018). Effects of long-term combination LT4 and LT3 therapy for improving hypothyroidism and overall quality of life. Southern medical journal, 111(6), 363.

32. Taroza, S., Rastenytė, D., Burkauskas, J., Podlipskytė, A., & Mickuvienė, N. (2019). Lower serum free triiodothyronine levels are associated with symptoms of depression after ischemic stroke. Journal of psychosomatic research, 122, 29-35.

33. Wang, K., Ojamaa, K., Samuels, A., Gilani, N., Zhang, K., An, S., ... & Gerdes, A. M. (2020). BNP as a new biomarker of cardiac thyroid hormone function. *Frontiers in physiology*, *11*, 729.

34. Weetman, A. P. (2021). An update on the pathogenesis of Hashimoto's thyroiditis. *Journal of endocrinological investigation*, *44*, 883-890.

35. Yamakawa, H., Kato, T. S., Noh, J. Y., Yuasa, S., Kawamura, A., Fukuda, K., & Aizawa, Y. (2021). Thyroid hormone plays an important role in cardiac function: from bench to bedside. *Frontiers in physiology*, *12*, 606931.

36. Yoon, B. H., Lee, Y., Oh, H. J., Kim, S. H., & Lee, Y. K. (2019). Influence of thyroid-stimulating hormone suppression therapy on bone mineral density in patients with differentiated thyroid cancer: a meta-analysis. Journal of bone metabolism, 26(1), 51-60.

37. https://www.tpauk.com/main/article/a-history-of-thyroid-treatments/

DHEA

1. Alexaki, V. I., Fodelianaki, G., Neuwirth, A., Mund, C., Kourgiantaki, A., Ieronimaki, E., ... & Chavakis, T. (2018). DHEA inhibits acute microglia-mediated inflammation through activation of the TrkA-Akt1/2-CREB-Jmjd3 pathway. *Molecular psychiatry*, *23*(6), 1410-1420.

2. Aly, H. F., Metwally, F. M., & Ahmed, H. H. (2011). Neuroprotective effects of dehydroepiandrosterone (DHEA) in rat model of Alzheimer's disease. *Acta Biochimica Polonica*, *58*(4).

3. Bentley, C., Hazeldine, J., Greig, C., Lord, J., & Foster, M. (2019). Dehydroepiandrosterone: a potential therapeutic agent in the treatment and rehabilitation of the traumatically injured patient. *Burns & trauma*, *7*.

4. Butcher, S. K., & Lord, J. M. (2004). Stress responses and innate immunity: aging as a contributory factor. *Aging cell*, *3*(4), 151-160.

5. Campbell, B. (2020). DHEAS and human development: An evolutionary perspective. *Frontiers in endocrinology*, *11*, 101

6. Corona, G., Rastrelli, G., Giagulli, V. A., Sila, A., Sforza, A., Forti, G., ... & Maggi, M. (2013). Dehydroepiandrosterone supplementation in elderly men: a meta-analysis study of placebo-controlled trials. *The Journal of Clinical Endocrinology & Metabolism*, *98*(9), 3615-3626

7. Fang, Y. H., Hsieh, M. J., Hung, M. S., Lin, Y. C., Kuo, L. T., Lu, M. L., ... & Chen, V. C. H. (2020). Low concentrations of dehydroepiandrosterone sulfate are associated with depression and fatigue in patients with non-small-cell lung cancer after chemotherapy. *Neuropsychiatric Disease and Treatment*, *16*, 2103.

8. Greaves, R. F., Wudy, S. A., Badoer, E., Zacharin, M., Hirst, J. J., Quinn, T., & Walker, D. W. (2019). A tale of two steroids: the importance of the androgens DHEA and DHEAS for early neurodevelopment. *The Journal of steroid biochemistry and molecular biology*, *188*, 77-85.

9. Hough, C. M., Lindqvist, D., Epel, E. S., Denis, M. S., Reus, V. I., Bersani, F. S., ... & Mellon, S. H. (2017). Higher serum DHEA concentrations before and after SSRI treatment are associated with remission of major depression. *Psychoneuroendocrinology*, *77*, 122-130.

10. Peixoto, C., Grande, A. J., Mallmann, M. B., Nardi, A. E., Cardoso, A., & Veras, A. B. (2018). Dehydroepiandrosterone (DHEA) for depression: a systematic review and meta-analysis. *CNS & Neurological Disorders-Drug Targets (Formerly Current Drug Targets-CNS & Neurological Disorders)*, *17*(9), 706-711.

11. Prall, S. P., Larson, E. E., & Muehlenbein, M. P. (2017). The role of dehydroepiandrosterone on functional innate immune responses to acute stress. *Stress and Health*, *33*(5), 656-664.

12. Rutkowski, K., Sowa, P., Rutkowska-Talipska, J., Kuryliszyn-Moskal, A., & Rutkowski, R. (2014). Dehydroepiandrosterone (DHEA): hypes and hopes. *Drugs*, *74*(11), 1195-1207.

13. Samaras, N., Samaras, D., Frangos, E., Forster, A., & Philippe, J. (2013). A review of age-related dehydroepiandrosterone decline and its association with well-known geriatric syndromes: is treatment beneficial?. *Rejuvenation research*, *16*(4), 285-294.

14. Savineau, J. P., Marthan, R., & de la Roque, E. D. (2013). Role of DHEA in cardiovascular diseases. *Biochemical pharmacology*, *85*(6), 718-726.

15. Souza-Teodoro, L. H., de Oliveira, C., Walters, K., & Carvalho, L. A. (2016). Higher serum dehydroepiandrosterone sulfate protects against the onset of depression in the elderly: findings from the English Longitudinal Study of Aging (ELSA). *Psychoneuroendocrinology, 64*, 40-46.Samaras, N., Samaras, D., Frangos, E., Forster, A., & Philippe, J. (2013). A review of age-related dehydroepiandrosterone decline and its association with well-known geriatric syndromes: is treatment beneficial?. *Rejuvenation research, 16*(4), 285-294.

16. Tipton, B. (2019). The Use of DHEA in the Treatment of Depression. PA Scholarly Poster Presentation University of Dakota.

17. Traish, A. M., Kang, H. P., Saad, F., & Guay, A. T. (2011). Dehydroepiandrosterone (DHEA)—a precursor steroid or an active hormone in human physiology (CME). The journal of sexual medicine, 8(11), 2960-2982.

18. Weiss, E. P., Shah, K., Fontana, L., Lambert, C. P., Holloszy, J. O., & Villareal, D. T. (2009). Dehydroepiandrosterone replacement therapy in older adults: 1-and 2-y effects on bone. *The American journal of clinical nutrition, 89*(5), 1459-1467.

19. Yanagita, I., Fujihara, Y., Kitajima, Y., Tajima, M., Honda, M., Kawajiri, T., ... & Muta, K. (2019). A high serum cortisol/DHEA-S ratio is a risk factor for sarcopenia in elderly diabetic patients. *Journal of the Endocrine Society, 3*(4), 801-813.

MELATONIN

1. Amaral, F. G. D., Andrade-Silva, J., Kuwabara, W. M., & Cipolla-Neto, J. (2019). New insights into the function of melatonin and its role in metabolic disturbances. *Expert review of endocrinology & metabolism, 14*(4), 293-300.

2. Baltatu, O. C., Amaral, F. G., Campos, L. A., & Cipolla-Neto, J. (2017). Melatonin, mitochondria and hypertension. *Cellular and molecular life sciences, 74*, 3955-3964.

3. Cipolla-Neto, J., Amaral, F. G., Soares Jr, J. M., Gallo, C. C., Furtado, A., Cavaco, J. E., ... & Quintela, T. (2022). The crosstalk between melatonin and sex steroid hormones. *Neuroendocrinology*, *112*(2), 115-129.

4. Favero, G., Franceschetti, L., Bonomini, F., Rodella, L. F., & Rezzani, R. (2017). Melatonin as an anti-inflammatory agent modulating inflammasome activation. *International journal of endocrinology*, *2017*.

5. González, A. G., Revilla, N. R., & Emilio, J. (2019). Clinical uses of melatonin: evaluation of human trials on cancer treatment. *Melatonin Research*, *2*(2), 47-69.

6. Kuwabara, W. M. T., Gomes, P. R. L., Andrade-Silva, J., Júnior, J. M. S., Amaral, F. G., & Cipolla-Neto, J. (2022). Melatonin and its ubiquitous effects on cell function and survival: A review. *Melatonin Research*, *5*(2), 192-208.

7. Mayo, J. C., Cernuda, R., Quiros, I., Rodriguez, P., Garcia, J. I., Hevia, D., & Sainz, R. M. (2019). Understanding the role of melatonin in cancer metabolism. *Melatonin Research*, *2*(3), 76-104.

8. Radogna, F., Diederich, M., & Ghibelli, L. (2010). Melatonin: a pleiotropic molecule regulating inflammation. *Biochemical pharmacology*, *80*(12), 1844-1852.

9. Reiter, R. J., Tan, D. X., Rosales-Corral, S., Galano, A., Zhou, X. J., & Xu, B. (2018). Mitochondria: central organelles for melatonin' s antioxidant and anti-aging actions. Molecules, 23(2), 509.

10. Tan, D. X., Manchester, L. C., Qin, L., & Reiter, R. J. (2016). Melatonin: a mitochondrial targeting molecule involving mitochondrial protection and dynamics. *International journal of molecular sciences*, *17*(12), 2124.

11. Tordjman, S., Chokron, S., Delorme, R., Charrier, A., Bellissant, E., Jaafari, N., & Fougerou, C. (2017). Melatonin: pharmacology, functions and therapeutic benefits. *Current neuropharmacology*, *15*(3), 434-443.

12. Wei, T., Li, C., Heng, Y., Gao, X., Zhang, G., Wang, H., ... & Hou, H. (2020). Association between night-shift work and level of melatonin: systematic review and meta-analysis. *Sleep medicine*, *75*, 502-509.

GUT HEALTH & NUTRIENT SUPPLEMENTS

1. Aguilera, M., Gálvez-Ontiveros, Y., & Rivas, A. (2020). Endobolome, a new concept for determining the influence of microbiota disrupting chemicals (MDC) in relation to specific endocrine pathogenesis. *Frontiers in Microbiology*, *11*, 578007.

2. Al-Rashidi, H. E. (2022). Gut microbiota and immunity relevance in eubiosis and dysbiosis. *Saudi Journal of Biological Sciences*, *29*(3), 1628-1643.

3. Amare, D. E. (2020). Anti-Cancer and Other Biological Effects of a Dietary Compound 3, 3□ -Diindolylmethane Supplementation: A Systematic Review of Human Clinical Trials. Nutrition and Dietary Supplements, 12, 123-137.

4. Amrein, K., Scherkl, M., Hoffmann, M., Neuwersch-Sommeregger, S., Köstenberger, M., Tmava Berisha, A., ... & Malle, O. (2020). Vitamin D deficiency 2.0: an update on the current status worldwide. *European journal of clinical nutrition*, *74*(11), 1498-1513.

5. Angelucci, F., Cechova, K., Amlerova, J., & Hort, J. (2019). Antibiotics, gut microbiota, and Alzheimer's disease. *Journal of neuroinflammation*, *16*(1), 1-10.

6. Atoum, M., & Alzoughool, F. (2017). Vitamin D and breast cancer: latest evidence and future steps. Breast cancer: basic and clinical research, 11, 1178223417749816.

7. Bajinka, O., Tan, Y., Abdelhalim, K. A., Özdemir, G., & Qiu, X. (2020). Extrinsic factors influencing gut microbes, the immediate consequences and restoring eubiosis. *AMB express*, *10*(1), 1-11.

8. Baker, J. M., Al-Nakkash, L., & Herbst-Kralovetz, M. M. (2017). Estrogen–gut microbiome axis: Physiological and clinical implications. *Maturitas*, *103*, 45-53.

9. Bajinka, O., Tan, Y., Abdelhalim, K. A., Özdemir, G., & Qiu, X. (2020). Extrinsic factors influencing gut microbes, the immediate consequences and restoring eubiosis. *AMB express*, *10*(1), 1-11.

10. Barandouzi, Z. A., Starkweather, A. R., Henderson, W. A., Gyamfi, A., & Cong, X. S. (2020). Altered composition of gut microbiota in depression: a systematic review. *Frontiers in psychiatry*, *11*, 541.

11. Benvenga, S., Ferrari, S. M., Elia, G., Ragusa, F., Patrizio, A., Paparo, S. R., ... & Fallahi, P. (2020). Nutraceuticals in thyroidology: A review of in vitro, and in vivo animal studies. *Nutrients*, *12*(5), 1337.

12. Benvenga, S., Feldt-Rasmussen, U., Bonofiglio, D., & Asamoah, E. (2019). Nutraceutical supplements in the thyroid setting: health benefits beyond basic nutrition. Nutrients, 11(9), 2214.

13. Bonofiglio, D., & Catalano, S. (2020). Effects of Iodine Intake and Nutraceuticals in Thyroidology: Update and Prospects. *Nutrients*, *12*(5), 1491.

14. Chandra, S., Sisodia, S. S., & Vassar, R. J. (2023). The gut microbiome in Alzheimer's disease: what we know and what remains to be explored. *Molecular neurodegeneration*, *18*(1), 1-21.

15. Chiovato, L., Magri, F., & Carlé, A. (2019). Hypothyroidism in context: where we've been and where we're going. *Advances in therapy*, *36*, 47-58.

16. Cheung, S. G., Goldenthal, A. R., Uhlemann, A. C., Mann, J. J., Miller, J. M., & Sublette, M. E. (2019). Systematic review of gut microbiota and major depression. *Frontiers in psychiatry*, *10*, 34.

17. Cho, J., Park, Y. J., Gonzales-Portillo, B., Saft, M., Cozene, B., Sadanandan, N., & Borlongan, C. V. (2021). Gut dysbiosis in stroke and its implications on Alzheimer's disease-like cognitive dysfunction. *CNS Neuroscience & Therapeutics,* 27(5), 505-514.

18. Calero-Medina, L., Jimenez-Casquet, M. J., Heras-Gonzalez, L., Conde-Pipo, J., Lopez-Moro, A., Olea-Serrano, F., & Mariscal-Arcas, M. (2023). Dietary exposure to endocrine disruptors in gut microbiota: A systematic review. *Science of the Total Environment*, 163991.

19. Coelho, L. J., & do Nascimento, G. N. L. (2020). Anti-inflammatory and diuretic activity of uncária tomentosa (cat's claw): systematic review. *Revista Cereus, 12*(2).

20. Cuenca-Micó, O., & Aceves, C. (2020). Micronutrients and Breast Cancer Progression: A Systematic Review. *Nutrients, 12*(12), 3613.

21. D'Andrea, S., Martorella, A., Coccia, F., Castellini, C., Minaldi, E., Totaro, M., ... & Barbonetti, A. (2021). Relationship of Vitamin D status with testosterone levels: a systematic review and meta-analysis. *Endocrine, 72*, 49-61.

22. De Cicco, P., Catani, M. V., Gasperi, V., Sibilano, M., Quaglietta, M., & Savini, I. (2019). Nutrition and breast cancer: a literature review on prevention, treatment and recurrence. *Nutrients, 11*(7), 1514.

23. Derry, D. (2001). Breast Cancer and iodine: How to prevent and survive breast cancer. Trafford.

24. Ervin, S. M., Li, H., Lim, L., Roberts, L. R., Liang, X., Mani, S., & Redinbo, M. R. (2019). Gut microbial β-glucuronidases reactivate estrogens as components of the estrobolome that reactivate estrogens. *Journal of Biological Chemistry, 294*(49), 18586-18599.

25. Filippone, A., Rossi, C., Rossi, M. M., Di Micco, A., Maggiore, C., Forcina, L., ... & Magno, S. (2023). Endocrine disruptors in food, estrobolome and breast cancer. *Journal of Clinical Medicine, 12*(9), 3158.

26. Gálvez-Ontiveros, Y., Páez, S., Monteagudo, C., & Rivas, A. (2020). Endocrine disruptors in food: impact on gut microbiota and metabolic diseases. *Nutrients, 12*(4), 1158.

27. Giau, V. V., Wu, S. Y., Jamerlan, A., An, S. S. A., Kim, S., & Hulme, J. (2018). Gut microbiota and their neuroinflammatory implications in Alzheimer's disease. *Nutrients, 10*(11), 1765.

28. Giuffrè, M., Moretti, R., Campisciano, G., da Silveira, A. B. M., Monda, V. M., Comar, M., ... & Crocè, L. S. (2020). You talking to me? Says the enteric nervous system (ENS) to the microbe. How intestinal microbes interact with the ENS. *Journal of Clinical Medicine, 9*(11), 3705.

29. Hall, D. (2001). Nutritional influences on estrogen metabolism. Applied nutritional science reports, 1, 1-8.

30. Hampl, R., & Stárka, L. (2020). Endocrine disruptors and gut microbiome interactions. *Physiological Research*, *69*(Suppl 2), S211.

31. Hiemstra, T. F., Lim, K., Thadhani, R., & Manson, J. E. (2019). Vitamin D and atherosclerotic cardiovascular disease. *The Journal of Clinical Endocrinology & Metabolism*, *104*(9), 4033-4050.

32. Hu, Y., Feng, W., Chen, H., Shi, H., Jiang, L., Zheng, X., ... & Cui, D. (2021). Effect of selenium on thyroid autoimmunity and regulatory T cells in patients with Hashimoto's thyroiditis: A prospective randomized-controlled trial. *Clinical and Translational Science,* 14(4), 1390-1402.

33. Hussain, T., Murtaza, G., Kalhoro, D. H., Kalhoro, M. S., Metwally, E., Chughtai, M. I., ... & Khan, S. A. (2021). Relationship between gut microbiota and host-metabolism: Emphasis on hormones related to reproductive function. *Animal Nutrition*, *7*(1), 1-10.

34. Illiano, P., Brambilla, R., & Parolini, C. (2020). The mutual interplay of gut microbiota, diet and human disease. *The FEBS journal*, *287*(5), 833-855.

35. Ihnatowicz, P., Drywień, M., Wątor, P., & Wojsiat, J. (2020). The importance of nutritional factors and dietary management of Hashimoto's thyroiditis. *Annals of agricultural and environmental medicine*, *27*(2), 184-193.

36. Insenser, M., Murri, M., Del Campo, R., Martinez-Garcia, M. A., Fernandez-Duran, E., & Escobar-Morreale, H. F. (2018). Gut microbiota and the polycystic ovary syndrome: influence of sex, sex hormones, and obesity. *The Journal of Clinical Endocrinology & Metabolism*, *103*(7), 2552-2562.

37. Kim, D. (2016). Low vitamin D status is associated with hypothyroid Hashimoto's thyroiditis. *Hormones*, *15*(3), 385-393.

38. Kinashi, Y., & Hase, K. (2021). Partners in leaky gut syndrome: intestinal dysbiosis and autoimmunity. *Frontiers in immunology*, *12*, 673708.

39. Kowalski, K., & Mulak, A. (2019). Brain-gut-microbiota axis in Alzheimer's disease. *Journal of neurogastroenterology and motility*, *25*(1), 48.

40. Latic, N., & Erben, R. G. (2020). Vitamin D and cardiovascular disease, with emphasis on hypertension, atherosclerosis, and heart failure. *International journal of molecular sciences*, *21*(18), 6483.

41. Lau, K., Srivatsav, V., Rizwan, A., Nashed, A., Liu, R., Shen, R., & Akhtar, M. (2017). Bridging the gap between gut microbial dysbiosis and cardiovascular diseases. *Nutrients*, *9*(8), 859.

42. Iebba, V., Totino, V., Gagliardi, A., Santangelo, F., Cacciotti, F., Trancassini, M., ... & Schippa, S. (2016). Eubiosis and dysbiosis: the two sides of the microbiota. *New Microbiol*, *39*(1), 1-12.

43. Lee, B. D., Yoo, J. M., Baek, S. Y., Li, F. Y., Sok, D. E., & Kim, M. R. (2020). 3, 3'-Diindolylmethane promotes BDNF and antioxidant enzyme formation via TrkB/Akt pathway activation for neuroprotection against oxidative stress-induced apoptosis in hippocampal neuronal cells. Antioxidants, 9(1), 3.

44. Li, J., Zhao, F., Wang, Y., Chen, J., Tao, J., Tian, G., ... & Cai, J. (2017). Gut microbiota dysbiosis contributes to the development of hypertension. *Microbiome*, *5*, 1-19.

45. Liu, S., Gao, J., Zhu, M., Liu, K., & Zhang, H. L. (2020). Gut microbiota and dysbiosis in Alzheimer's disease: implications for pathogenesis and treatment. *Molecular neurobiology*, *57*, 5026-5043.

46. Lobionda, S., Sittipo, P., Kwon, H. Y., & Lee, Y. K. (2019). The role of gut microbiota in intestinal inflammation with respect to diet and extrinsic stressors. *Microorganisms*, *7*(8), 271.

47. Luo, Q., Yang, A., Cao, Q., & Guan, H. (2018). 3, 3'-Diindolylmethane

protects cardiomyocytes from LPS-induced inflammatory response and apoptosis. BMC Pharmacology and Toxicology, 19(1), 1-9.

48. Margolis, K. G., Cryan, J. F., & Mayer, E. A. (2021). The microbiota-gut-brain axis: from motility to mood. *Gastroenterology*, *160*(5), 1486-1501.

49. Maffei, S., Forini, F., Canale, P., Nicolini, G., & Guiducci, L. (2022). Gut microbiota and sex hormones: crosstalking players in cardiometabolic and cardiovascular disease. *International Journal of Molecular Sciences*, *23*(13), 7154.

50. Manjer, J., Sandsveden, M., & Borgquist, S. (2020). Serum Iodine and Breast Cancer Risk: A Prospective Nested Case–Control Study Stratified for Selenium Levels. *Cancer Epidemiology, Biomarkers & Prevention*, *29*(7), 1335-1340.

51. Marietta, E., Horwath, I., Balakrishnan, B., & Taneja, V. (2019). Role of the intestinal microbiome in autoimmune diseases and its use in treatments. *Cellular immunology*, 339, 50-58.

52. Michos, E. D., Cainzos-Achirica, M., Heravi, A. S., & Appel, L. J. (2021). Vitamin D, calcium supplements, and implications for cardiovascular health: JACC focus seminar. *Journal of the American College of Cardiology*, *77*(4), 437-449.

53. Mokbel, K., & Mokbel, K. (2019). Chemoprevention of breast cancer with vitamins and micronutrients: A concise review. *in vivo*, *33*(4), 983-997.

54. Monneret, C. (2017). What is an endocrine disruptor?. *Comptes rendus biologies*, *340*(9-10), 403-405.

55. Morais, L. H., Schreiber IV, H. L., & Mazmanian, S. K. (2021). The gut microbiota–brain axis in behaviour and brain disorders. *Nature Reviews Microbiology*, *19*(4), 241-255.

56. Mu, Q., Kirby, J., Reilly, C. M., & Luo, X. M. (2017). Leaky gut as a danger signal for autoimmune diseases. *Frontiers in immunology*, 598.

57. Nimptsch, K., Platz, E. A., Willett, W. C., & Giovannucci, E. (2012). Association between plasma 25-OH vitamin D and testosterone levels in men. Clinical endocrinology, 77(1), 106-112.

58. Osowiecka, K., & Myszkowska-Ryciak, J. (2023). The Influence of Nutritional Intervention in the Treatment of Hashimoto's Thyroiditis—A Systematic Review. *Nutrients, 15*(4), 1041.

59. Paray, B. A., Albeshr, M. F., Jan, A. T., & Rather, I. A. (2020). Leaky gut and autoimmunity: an intricate balance in individuals health and the diseased state. *International journal of molecular sciences, 21*(24), 9770.

60. Parkin, K., Christophersen, C. T., Verhasselt, V., Cooper, M. N., & Martino, D. (2021). Risk factors for gut dysbiosis in early life. *Microorganisms*, 9(10), 2066.

61. Pilz, S., Verheyen, N., Grübler, M. R., Tomaschitz, A., & März, W. (2016). Vitamin D and cardiovascular disease prevention. *Nature Reviews Cardiology, 13*(7), 404-417.

62. Qi, X., Yun, C., Pang, Y., & Qiao, J. (2021). The impact of the gut microbiota on the reproductive and metabolic endocrine system. *Gut Microbes, 13*(1), 1894070.

63. Regal, P., Fente, C. A., Cepeda, A., & Silva, E. G. (2021). Food and omics: unraveling the role of food in breast cancer development. *Current Opinion in Food Science, 39*, 197-207.

64. Rheaume-Bleue, K. (2011). Vitamin K2 and the calcium paradox: how a little-known vitamin could save your life. John Wiley & Sons.

65. Rostami, R., Nourooz-Zadeh, S., Mohammadi, A., Khalkhali, H. R., Ferns, G., & Nourooz-Zadeh, J. (2020). Serum selenium status and its interrelationship with serum biomarkers of thyroid function and antioxidant defense in Hashimoto's thyroiditis. *Antioxidants, 9*(11), 1070.

66. Ruo, S. W., Alkayyali, T., Win, M., Tara, A., Joseph, C., Kannan, A., ... & Poudel, S. (2021). Role of gut microbiota dysbiosis in breast cancer and novel approaches in prevention, diagnosis, and treatment. *Cureus, 13*(8).

67. Simpson, C. A., Diaz-Arteche, C., Eliby, D., Schwartz, O. S., Simmons, J. G., & Cowan, C. S. (2021). The gut microbiota in anxiety and depression–a systematic review. *Clinical psychology review*, *83*, 101943.

68. Singhvi, N., Gupta, V., Gaur, M., Sharma, V., Puri, A., Singh, Y., ... & Lal, R. (2020). Interplay of human gut microbiome in health and wellness. *Indian journal of microbiology*, *60*, 26-36.

69. Sharma, R., Bharti, S., & Kumar, K. H. (2014). Diet and thyroid-myths and facts. *Journal of Medical Nutrition and Nutraceuticals*, *3*(2), 60.

70. Sofianopoulou, E., Kaptoge, S. K., Afzal, S., Jiang, T., Gill, D., Gundersen, T. E., ... & Burgess, S. (2021). Estimating dose-response relationships for vitamin D with coronary heart disease, stroke, and all-cause mortality: observational and Mendelian randomisation analyses. *The Lancet Diabetes & Endocrinology*, *9*(12), 837-846.

71. Suparan, K., Sriwichaiin, S., Chattipakorn, N., & Chattipakorn, S. C. (2022). Human Blood Bacteriome: Eubiotic and Dysbiotic States in Health and Diseases. *Cells*, *11*(13), 2015.

72. Sordi, R., Castro, S. N., Lera, A. T., Irene, M. N., Farinazzo, M. D. M., Sette, C., ... & Del Giglio, A. (2019). Randomized, double-blind, placebo-controlled phase ii clinical trial on the use of uncaria tomentosa (Cat's claw) for aromatase inhibitor-induced arthralgia: a pilot study. *Journal of Natural Remedies*, *19*(1), 24-31.

73. Sui, Y., Wu, J., & Chen, J. (2021). The role of gut microbial β-glucuronidase in estrogen reactivation and breast cancer. *Frontiers in cell and developmental biology*, *9*, 631552.

74. Thomson, C. A., Chow, H. S., Wertheim, B. C., Roe, D. J., Stopeck, A., Maskarinec, G., ... & Thompson, P. A. (2017). A randomized, placebo-controlled trial of diindolylmethane for breast cancer biomarker modulation in patients taking tamoxifen. Breast cancer research and treatment, 165(1), 97-107.

75. Triggiani, V., Tafaro, E., Giagulli, V. A., Sabbà, C., Resta, F., Licchelli, B., & Guastamacchia, E. (2009). Role of iodine, selenium and other

micronutrients in thyroid function and disorders. *Endocrine, Metabolic & Immune Disorders-Drug Targets (Formerly Current Drug Targets-Immune, Endocrine & Metabolic Disorders)*, *9*(3), 277-294.

76. Valles-Colomer, M., Falony, G., Darzi, Y., Tigchelaar, E. F., Wang, J., Tito, R. Y., ... & Raes, J. (2019). The neuroactive potential of the human gut microbiota in quality of life and depression. *Nature microbiology*, *4*(4), 623-632.

77. Varesi, A., Pierella, E., Romeo, M., Piccini, G. B., Alfano, C., Bjørklund, G., ... & Pascale, A. (2022). The potential role of gut microbiota in Alzheimer's disease: From diagnosis to treatment. *Nutrients*, *14*(3), 668.

78. Vranić, L., Mikolašević, I., & Milić, S. (2019). Vitamin D deficiency: consequence or cause of obesity?. *Medicina*, *55*(9), 541.

79. Wu, W. J. H., Zegarra-Ruiz, D. F., & Diehl, G. E. (2020). Intestinal microbes in autoimmune and inflammatory disease. *Frontiers in Immunology*, *11*, 597966.

80. Yepes-Pérez, A. F., Herrera-Calderon, O., & Quintero-Saumeth, J. (2022). Uncaria tomentosa (cat's claw): a promising herbal medicine against SARS-CoV-2/ACE-2 junction and SARS-CoV-2 spike protein based on molecular modeling. *Journal of Biomolecular Structure and Dynamics*, *40*(5), 2227-2243.

81. Yerushalmi, R., Bargil, S., Ber, Y., Ozlavo, R., Sivan, T., Rapson, Y., ... & Margel, D. (2020). 3, 3-Diindolylmethane (DIM): a nutritional intervention and its impact on breast density in healthy BRCA carriers. A prospective clinical trial. Carcinogenesis, 41(10), 1395-1401.

82. Zheng, D., Liao, H., Chen, S., Liu, X., Mao, C., Zhang, C., ... & Chen, Y. (2021). Elevated levels of circulating biomarkers related to leaky gut syndrome and bacterial translocation are associated with graves' disease. *Frontiers in endocrinology*, *12*, 796212.

RESOURCES

1. Network of providers trained in the art and science of hormone optimization: www.evexias.com
2. Metabolic Code information: www.metaboliccode.com
3. Life changing coaching and content: Think Differently Academy www.tdacad.com

ABOUT THE AUTHOR

Terri DeNeui, DNP, APRN, ACNP-BC

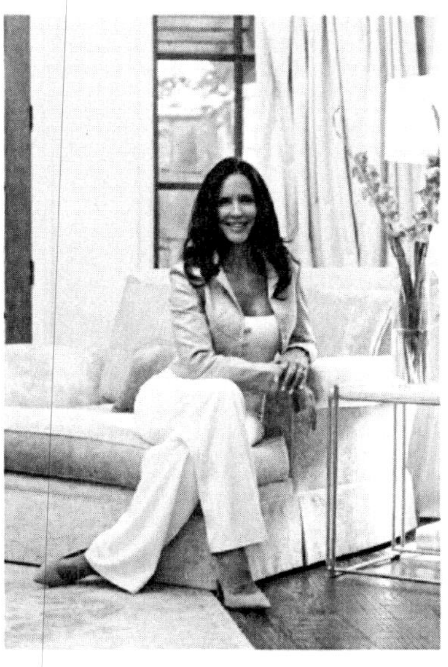

Terri DeNeui, DNP, APRN, ACNP-BC is the founder of EVEXIAS Health Solutions and creator of the EvexiPEL Method. She leads the EVEXIAS Medical Advisory Board, hand selecting leading experts from around the globe to support the education and knowledge resources that provide the opportunity to experience a whole new way to practice medicine that is truly transformational for patients and practitioners.

Dr. Terri DeNeui is a board-certified nurse practitioner, nationally renowned speaker, author, and entrepreneur. She holds advanced certifications in Hormone Replacement Therapy, Preventive Wellness Medicine, and Functional Medicine. Dr. DeNeui earned her bachelor's degree in nursing from Texas Women's University, and achieved both her master's and doctorate degrees in nursing from the University of Texas at Arlington.

Her career in medicine began as a hospitalist in emergency medicine, where Dr. DeNeui quickly realized that day in and day out, the focus was on disease management instead of disease prevention. She felt saddened and frustrated—she wanted to do more for patient care and for that, she had to know more.

This was the catalyst for what is now her life's work. She began to pursue extensive education in hormone optimization, integrative health, preventive care, and alternative medicine. It was in a lecture by physician and author of Awakening Athena, Dr. Kenna Stephenson, that she knew hormone therapy and integrative medicine pursuits would be how she would spend her career.

Dr. DeNeui founded Hormonal Health & Wellness in Southlake, Texas (now EVEXIAS Medical Centers) in 2008 as the first step in her new pursuit. In her practice, Dr. DeNeui strives to help men and women find optimal health. Her success and the positive outcomes that her patients enjoy can be attributed to her thirst for knowledge. She says, "I will never stop asking questions. I will never stop seeking answers. If a patient is not achieving optimal results, we must ask more questions and uncover answers—sometimes answers we didn't know were there when we first asked the question. Medicine and science are ever evolving. We can never stop asking questions or seeking answers."

That thirst for knowledge led her to discover pellet therapy and the benefits of testosterone in women. Fifteen years ago, she traveled to Arizona to train with Gino Tutera, one of the pioneers of hormone pellet therapy. Her experience there led her to introduce pellet therapy into her practice and evolve her treatment methods. In a few short years, her methodology became renowned, evolving into a brand known today as the EvexiPEL Method. To date, thousands of practitioners have been trained and certified in the EvexiPEL Method and tens of thousands of patients are living happier, healthier, and better lives because of EvexiPEL.

In 2018, she partnered with researchers, pharmacists, and scientists at FarmaKeio Outsourcing, an FDA-registered outsourcing facility, to develop a proprietary pellet formulation. The pellet is has since become recognized for its uniqueness and received a U.S. patent in 2023.

When describing her hopes for her patients, Dr. DeNeui says, “At EVEXIAS, we believe in an integrated approach to wellness that includes not only education, but evaluation of the individual patient as a whole rather than just a specific problem that he or she may present.”

When she’s not seeing patients, Dr. DeNeui loves to spend time with her husband, their two dogs, their seven children, and four grandchildren. She also enjoys traveling anywhere near the water, drinking wine, reading books, and continuously researching.

ABOUT EVEXIAS HEALTH SOLUTIONS

EVEXIAS Health Solutions is an emerging leader in the advancement of medicine toward a preventive care model that positively impacts the lives of patients and practitioners.

The EVEXIAS team has helped thousands of practitioners across the nation enhance patient care and expand their treatment plans through advanced medical education and training from industry-leading medical practitioners, researchers, and scientists, as well as providing access to leading-edge therapies and technologies that support the prevention of disease and improve quality of life. Every EHS program is backed by strategic business plans and operational practices exclusively developed for private medical practices to achieve the highest level of patient experience and outcomes for the practices served.

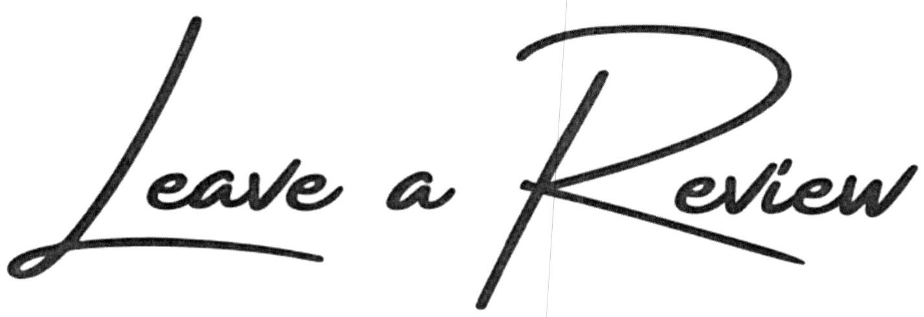

Love the book?

Scan the QR Code below to share your experience.

FORWARD BY KELLY LEBROCK

HORMONE Havoc

Dispelling the Myths & Misconceptions about Hormones in Women & Men

Dr. Terri DeNeui
DNP, APRN, ACNP-BC

Leave a Review

HORMONEHAVOC.COM

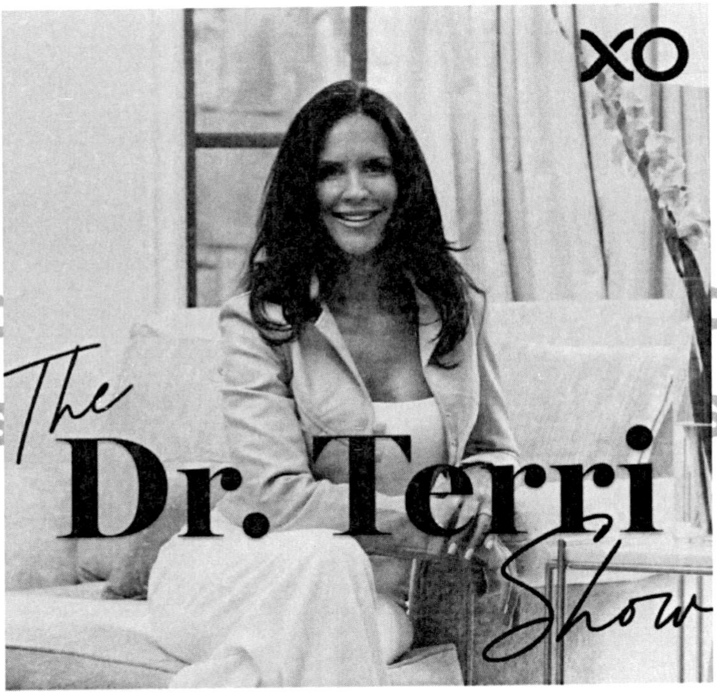

The Dr. Terri Show

Are you sick and tired of feeling sick and tired? Do you desire to live a life of abundance in your health? On the Dr. Terri Show, we cut through all of the hype and fads to bring you real, vulnerable conversations about health, faith, and life.

Listen on
Apple Podcasts

Listen on
Spotify Podcasts